DIABETES TEA RECIPES

Tapping Into The Restorative Power of Nature for Blood Sugar Control and Wellness

By

Hector Wiggins

Table of Contents

INTRODUCTION

In a world where chronic diseases like diabetes are on the rise, the quest for natural remedies and holistic approaches to health has never been more urgent. Welcome to **"Diabetes Tea Recipes:** Harnessing the Healing Power of Nature for Blood Sugar Control and Wellness." Within the pages of this comprehensive guide, we embark on a journey of discovery, exploring the profound connection between herbal teas and the management of diabetes.

Understanding Diabetes:
Diabetes, a metabolic disorder characterized by high levels of glucose in the blood, affects millions of individuals worldwide. Type 1 diabetes, typically diagnosed in childhood or adolescence, results from the body's inability to produce insulin, the hormone responsible for regulating blood sugar levels.

On the other hand, type 2 diabetes, the most common form of the disease, occurs when the body becomes resistant to insulin or fails to produce enough of it. Gestational diabetes, which develops during pregnancy, presents unique challenges for expectant mothers and requires careful monitoring.

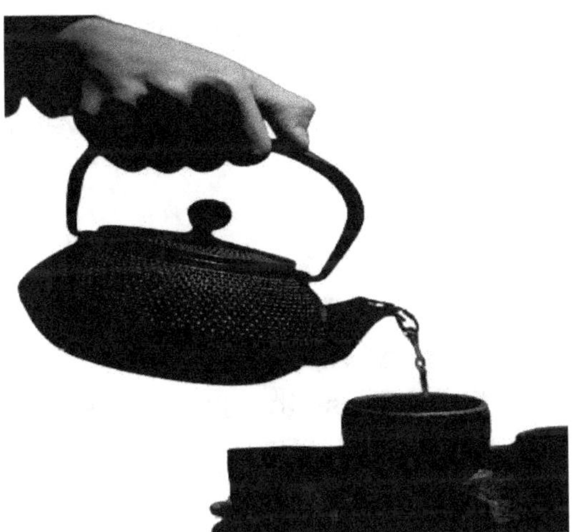

The Role of Herbal Teas:
Amidst the complexity of diabetes management, herbal teas emerge as a beacon of hope, offering natural solutions to support blood sugar control and overall wellness. For centuries, cultures around the world have revered herbal infusions for their medicinal properties and therapeutic benefits. From traditional remedies passed down through generations to modern scientific discoveries, the healing power of tea continues to captivate and inspire.

Empowering Through Recipes:
In "Diabetes Tea Recipes," we present a diverse collection of herbal tea recipes carefully curated to address the specific needs of individuals living with diabetes.

Each recipe is crafted with intention, combining the finest herbs, spices, and botanicals known for their ability to support blood sugar regulation, improve insulin sensitivity, and alleviate diabetic symptoms.

Exploring the Chapters:
The journey begins with a deeper understanding of diabetes and its management strategies in Chapter 1. Subsequent chapters delve into the benefits of tea for diabetes management, exploring the science behind herbal remedies and their impact on blood sugar control. From herbal infusions and green tea varieties to spice-infused elixirs and antioxidant-rich blends, each chapter offers a unique perspective on harnessing the healing power of nature.

Beyond the Cup:

But "Diabetes Tea Recipes" is more than just a collection of beverages; it's a guide to embracing a holistic approach to diabetes wellness. Throughout the book, we emphasize the importance of mindful tea drinking practices, stress management techniques, and incorporating tea into a balanced lifestyle. By embracing holistic approaches such as mindfulness, meditation, and yoga, individuals can cultivate resilience, reduce stress, and enhance their overall quality of life.

Understanding the Impact of Tea on Diabetes Management

Tea, a beloved beverage enjoyed by millions worldwide, holds immense potential as a natural remedy for managing diabetes. In this chapter, we delve into the profound impact of tea on diabetes management, exploring its role in blood sugar regulation, insulin sensitivity, and overall health and wellness.

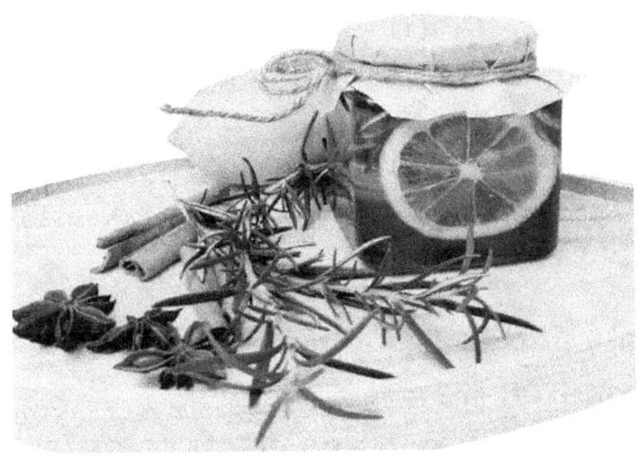

The Science Behind Tea and Blood Sugar Regulation:

Numerous studies have highlighted the beneficial effects of tea consumption on blood sugar levels. Tea, derived from the Camellia plant and various herbs, contains bioactive compounds such as polyphenols and antioxidants that play a key role in regulating glucose metabolism. Polyphenols, including catechins and flavonoids, exhibit anti-inflammatory and antioxidant properties, which may help improve insulin sensitivity and reduce insulin resistance. Additionally, the caffeine content in tea has been shown to enhance glucose uptake and utilization by skeletal muscles, further contributing to improved blood sugar control.

Antioxidants and Polyphenols: Their Role in **Diabetes Control:**

One of the most notable components of tea is its high antioxidant content.

Antioxidants help neutralize harmful free radicals in the body, which can contribute to oxidative stress and inflammation, both of which are implicated in the development and progression of diabetes. Polyphenols, a type of antioxidant found abundantly in tea, have been extensively studied for their potential therapeutic effects on diabetes. These compounds may help protect pancreatic beta cells, which are responsible for producing insulin, from damage caused by oxidative stress, thus preserving their function and promoting insulin secretion.

How Tea Consumption Can Support Overall Health in Diabetes:
Beyond its direct effects on blood sugar regulation, tea consumption offers a myriad of additional health benefits that can be particularly beneficial for individuals with diabetes.

Regular tea consumption has been associated with reduced risk of cardiovascular disease, which is a major complication of diabetes. The anti-inflammatory properties of tea may help alleviate inflammation in blood vessels, improve endothelial function, and reduce the risk of atherosclerosis and heart disease. Furthermore, tea's potential to lower blood pressure and improve lipid profile adds to its cardioprotective effects, making it a valuable addition to a diabetes-friendly diet.

Conclusion:

In conclusion, the impact of tea on diabetes management extends far beyond its comforting aroma and soothing taste. From its ability to regulate blood sugar levels and improve insulin sensitivity to its potent antioxidant properties and cardiovascular benefits, tea stands as a powerful ally in the fight against diabetes.

By incorporating a variety of herbal teas and green tea infusions into your daily routine, you can harness the healing power of nature to support your journey towards better blood sugar control and overall wellness. In the following chapters, we'll explore a range of delicious tea recipes specifically tailored to support individuals with diabetes, providing you with a diverse array of options to enhance your health and well-being.

The Role of Herbal Teas in Blood Sugar Control

In the realm of managing diabetes, the quest for effective, natural remedies is ceaseless. Herbal teas have emerged as a popular option, offering not just warmth and comfort but also potential benefits in blood sugar control. These "diabetes tea recipes" harness the power of various herbs, each with its unique properties that may aid in managing blood glucose levels.

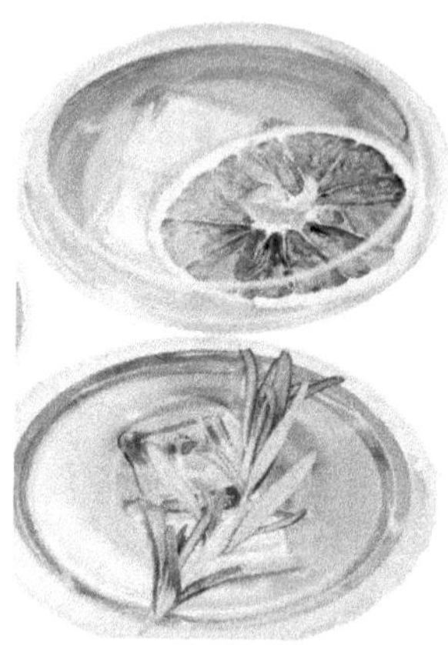

Cinnamon Tea: Cinnamon, a staple spice in many cuisines, is also celebrated for its potential in diabetes management. Its active compound, cinnamaldehyde, has been studied for its insulin-like effects. Brewing a simple cinnamon tea by steeping cinnamon sticks or powder in hot water can be a soothing and potentially beneficial addition to a diabetic's routine.

Ginger Tea: Ginger, renowned for its anti-inflammatory and antioxidant properties, may also offer benefits in glycemic control. Studies suggest that ginger may improve insulin sensitivity and reduce fasting blood sugar levels. Brewing ginger tea by simmering fresh ginger slices in water can create a flavorful and healthful beverage for diabetes management.

Fenugreek Tea: Fenugreek seeds have a long history of use in traditional medicine for various ailments, including diabetes. Rich in soluble fiber, fenugreek may help slow down the absorption of sugar and improve insulin sensitivity. To make fenugreek tea, steep fenugreek seeds in hot water and strain before drinking for a potentially beneficial addition to a diabetic diet.

Tea made from holy basil: Known by another name, tulsi, holy basil is highly valued in Ayurveda for its therapeutic qualities. By enhancing glucose absorption and promoting insulin secretion, it might assist in lowering blood sugar levels. Making holy basil tea from dried or fresh leaves can be a relaxing and possibly helpful drink for those who have diabetes.

Green Tea:
Green tea, cherished for its numerous health benefits, also shows promise in blood sugar control. Its high concentration of polyphenols, particularly epigallocatechin gallate (EGCG), may enhance insulin sensitivity and reduce blood sugar levels. Enjoying a cup of green tea regularly can be a refreshing and healthful habit for diabetes management.

How This Book Can Help You

In the world of diabetes management, exploring natural remedies can be empowering and enlightening. "Diabetes Tea Recipes" offers a unique approach by introducing a collection of herbal tea recipes specifically curated to aid in blood sugar control. This book serves as a valuable resource for individuals seeking alternative and complementary methods to manage their diabetes effectively.

Understanding Herbal Teas and Diabetes: Before delving into the recipes, this book provides a comprehensive overview of herbal teas and their potential benefits for individuals with diabetes. It explores the science behind various herbs and their effects on blood sugar levels, empowering readers with knowledge to make informed choices.

A Variety of Recipes for Every Palate:
From soothing cinnamon tea to invigorating
ginger tea, this book presents a diverse array
of recipes to suit every taste preference. Each
recipe is carefully crafted to not only tantalize
the taste buds but also provide potential
benefits in glycemic control, offering readers a
delightful and healthful beverage option.

Easy-to-Follow Instructions and Tips:
Whether you're a seasoned tea aficionado or
new to the world of herbal remedies, this book
ensures accessibility with clear and concise
instructions for each recipe. Additionally, it
offers helpful tips and suggestions for
ingredient substitutions or variations, allowing
readers to customize the recipes to their liking.

Embracing Tradition and Innovation:
Drawing inspiration from both traditional
wisdom and modern research, "Diabetes Tea
Recipes" combines time-honored herbal
remedies with contemporary culinary
innovation.

It celebrates the rich heritage of herbal medicine while embracing the latest findings in diabetes management, offering readers a holistic and dynamic approach to wellness.

Empowerment Through Self-Care:
Beyond just providing recipes, this book encourages readers to embrace self-care and mindfulness in their diabetes management journey. Brewing and savoring a cup of herbal tea can become a ritual of self-love and nourishment, fostering a deeper connection with one's health and well-being.

Complementary to Conventional Treatment:
While herbal teas can offer potential benefits in blood sugar control, this book emphasizes the importance of integrating them into a comprehensive diabetes management plan. It underscores the complementary nature of herbal remedies alongside conventional treatments, advocating for a holistic approach to wellness.

Expert Insights and Recommendations:
Backed by expert insights and recommendations, "Diabetes Tea Recipes" ensures credibility and reliability in its content. It draws upon the expertise of healthcare professionals, herbalists, and nutritionists to provide readers with evidence-based guidance and support in their journey towards better health.

"Diabetes Tea Recipes" is more than just a collection of beverages; it's a guidebook for holistic diabetes management and well-being. By embracing the power of herbal teas, readers can embark on a journey of self-discovery and empowerment, taking proactive steps towards better health and vitality. With its wealth of knowledge, accessible recipes, and expert guidance, this book equips readers with the tools they need to thrive in their diabetes management journey.

CHAPTER ONE

Understanding Diabetes and Its Management

High blood glucose levels are a hallmark of diabetes, a chronic illness brought on by either insufficient or inefficient insulin synthesis or utilization by the body. Maintaining general health and preventing complications from diabetes require effective treatment. While medicine, food, and exercise are the mainstays of standard treatment, investigating supplementary methods like herbal teas can help improve blood sugar management even more.

Comprehending Diabetes: Diabetes is a collection of metabolic conditions that impact the way the body utilizes glucose, or blood sugar. Insulin insufficiency is the outcome of the immune system targeting the pancreatic beta cells that produce insulin in type 1 diabetes. When the body either stops producing enough insulin to maintain normal glucose levels or becomes resistant to insulin, type 2 diabetes develops.

The Importance of Blood Sugar Control: Managing blood sugar levels is essential for individuals with diabetes to prevent complications such as heart disease, kidney damage, nerve damage, and vision problems. Consistent monitoring and maintenance of blood glucose levels within target ranges are vital to reduce the risk of long-term complications.

Conventional Diabetes Management: Conventional diabetes management typically involves a combination of medication, lifestyle modifications, and regular monitoring of blood sugar levels.

Medications may include insulin injections, oral medications to lower blood sugar, or other drugs to manage associated conditions such as high blood pressure and cholesterol.

The Role of Herbal Teas:
Herbal teas have gained popularity for their potential health benefits, including aiding in blood sugar control. Certain herbs and spices contain compounds that may improve insulin sensitivity, promote glucose metabolism, and reduce inflammation, making them valuable additions to a diabetic diet.

Benefits of Herbal Teas in Diabetes Management:

Cinnamon: Contains compounds that mimic the effects of insulin and may help lower blood sugar levels.

Ginger: Known for its anti-inflammatory properties, ginger may improve insulin sensitivity and reduce fasting blood sugar levels.

Fenugreek: Rich in soluble fiber, fenugreek seeds may help slow down the absorption of sugar and improve insulin sensitivity.

Holy Basil: Stimulates insulin secretion and may help lower blood sugar levels.

Antioxidants found in green tea may improve insulin sensitivity and lower blood sugar levels. Including Herbal Teas in a Plan for Diabetes Management:

While herbal teas can offer potential benefits in blood sugar control, it's important to integrate them into a comprehensive diabetes management plan.

Herbal teas should complement, not replace, conventional treatments prescribed by healthcare professionals. Regular monitoring of blood sugar levels is essential to assess the effectiveness of herbal remedies.

"Diabetes Tea Recipes" provides a holistic approach to diabetes management by incorporating the benefits of herbal teas into daily routines. By understanding diabetes and the role of herbal remedies in blood sugar control, individuals can make informed choices to enhance their overall well-being. With a combination of conventional treatments, lifestyle modifications, and the inclusion of healthful herbal teas, individuals with diabetes can take proactive steps towards managing their condition effectively and improving their quality of life.

Types of Diabetes: Type 1, Type 2, Gestational Diabetes

A complicated metabolic disease with high blood sugar levels is called diabetes. It is essential to comprehend the many forms of diabetes in order to manage and treat it effectively. Every kind of diabetes, including gestational diabetes and Types 1 and 2, has its own set of issues and concerns. Even though traditional therapies are important, trying complementary methods like herbal teas might help manage the illness even more.

Type 1 Diabetes: Also referred to as insulin-dependent diabetes or juvenile diabetes, type 1 diabetes is caused by an immune system error that causes the pancreatic beta cells that produce insulin to be attacked and destroyed. Insulin production is reduced or nonexistent as a result, necessitating daily insulin injections for survival. Although it can strike at any age, type 1 diabetes usually appears in childhood or adolescence. Blood sugar monitoring, insulin medication, and a balanced diet are all part of management.

Type 2 Diabetes: With the majority of instances occurring globally, type 2 diabetes is the most prevalent type of the disease. It happens when the body stops producing enough insulin to keep blood sugar levels within normal ranges or develops resistance to insulin. Poor food choices, physical inactivity, and obesity are among the lifestyle factors that are frequently associated with type 2 diabetes. Medications taken orally, insulin therapy, diet and exercise changes, and routine blood sugar testing are examples of management techniques.

Gestational Diabetes: When the body cannot manufacture enough insulin to satisfy the increasing demands, gestational diabetes develops during pregnancy. It normally goes away after labor and manifests in the second or third trimester. On the other hand, women who acquire gestational diabetes have a higher chance of acquiring Type 2 diabetes in the future. In order to maintain a healthy pregnancy and avoid difficulties for the woman and the unborn child, management strategies include blood sugar monitoring, dietary modifications, exercise, and occasionally insulin therapy.

Exploring Herbal Tea Support:
While conventional treatments are essential for managing all types of diabetes, incorporating herbal teas into a diabetes management plan can provide additional support. Certain herbs and spices found in herbal teas have been studied for their potential benefits in blood sugar control and insulin sensitivity.

From cinnamon and ginger to fenugreek and green tea, these natural remedies offer a flavorful and healthful way to complement traditional treatments.

"Diabetes Tea Recipes" sheds light on the diverse landscape of diabetes, encompassing Type 1, Type 2, and gestational diabetes. By understanding the unique characteristics and management strategies associated with each type, individuals can take proactive steps towards better health and well-being. While conventional treatments remain the cornerstone of diabetes management, the inclusion of herbal teas offers an additional avenue for support and exploration. With a holistic approach that embraces both traditional wisdom and modern science, individuals with diabetes can navigate their journey with confidence and empowerment.

Symptoms and Complications of Diabetes

Recognizing the symptoms of diabetes and understanding its potential complications are crucial for early detection, effective management, and prevention of long-term health issues. While conventional treatments play a significant role in controlling diabetes, exploring complementary approaches like herbal teas can offer additional support in mitigating symptoms and reducing the risk of complications.

Symptoms of Diabetes:

Frequent Urination (Polyuria): Excess glucose in the bloodstream leads to increased urine production, causing frequent urination.

Excessive Thirst (Polydipsia): Dehydration resulting from frequent urination triggers feelings of thirst.

Unexplained Weight Loss: Despite increased appetite and food intake, individuals may experience unexplained weight loss due to the body's inability to use glucose for energy.

Fatigue: Insufficient glucose uptake by cells leads to fatigue and weakness, as cells lack the energy needed to function properly.

Blurry Vision: High blood sugar levels can cause changes in the shape of the lens in the eye, leading to blurry vision.

Slow Healing of Wounds: Elevated blood sugar levels impair the body's ability to heal wounds and injuries efficiently.

Complications of Diabetes:

Cardiovascular Disease: Diabetes significantly increases the risk of heart disease, stroke, and peripheral artery disease due to the impact of high blood sugar levels on blood vessels and circulation.

Kidney Disease (Nephropathy): Diabetes is a leading cause of kidney failure, as high blood sugar levels over time damage the kidneys' filtering units.

Nerve Damage (Neuropathy): Elevated blood sugar levels can cause nerve damage, resulting in pain, tingling, numbness, or loss of sensation, particularly in the extremities.

Eye Damage (Retinopathy): Diabetes can lead to damage to the blood vessels in the retina, potentially causing vision loss or blindness if left untreated.

Foot Complications: Poor circulation and nerve damage increase the risk of foot ulcers, infections, and even amputations in individuals with diabetes.

Skin Conditions: Diabetes can increase the risk of various skin conditions, including bacterial and fungal infections, as well as diabetic dermopathy and acanthosis nigricans.

Herbal Teas for Symptom Management and Prevention:

While herbal teas cannot cure diabetes or its complications, certain herbs and spices found in herbal teas may help alleviate symptoms and reduce the risk of complications.

For example, cinnamon tea may help regulate blood sugar levels, ginger tea may reduce inflammation and improve circulation, and green tea may offer antioxidant protection against cardiovascular disease.

Holy basil tea and fenugreek tea are also believed to have potential benefits in blood sugar control and may help mitigate some of the symptoms associated with diabetes.

Strategies for Managing Diabetes: Blood Sugar Monitoring, Healthy Eating, Exercise, Medication

Managing diabetes effectively requires a multifaceted approach that includes blood sugar monitoring, healthy eating, regular exercise, and medication as necessary. While these strategies form the foundation of diabetes management, incorporating complementary approaches like herbal teas can provide additional support and contribute to overall well-being.

Blood Sugar Monitoring:
Regular blood sugar monitoring is essential for individuals with diabetes to track their glucose levels and make informed decisions about medication, diet, and lifestyle.

Monitoring techniques include self-monitoring of blood glucose (using a glucometer), continuous glucose monitoring (CGM) systems, and periodic A1C testing to assess long-term blood sugar control.

Healthy Eating:
A balanced and nutritious diet is crucial for managing blood sugar levels and preventing complications associated with diabetes.
Focus on consuming whole foods, including plenty of fruits, vegetables, lean proteins, and whole grains, while limiting processed foods, sugary beverages, and high-fat foods.
Herbal teas, such as cinnamon tea and green tea, can complement a healthy diet by providing antioxidants and potential benefits in blood sugar control.

Regular Exercise:
Physical activity plays a key role in diabetes management by improving insulin sensitivity, lowering blood sugar levels, and supporting overall cardiovascular health.

Aim for at least 150 minutes of
moderate-intensity aerobic exercise per week,
along with strength training exercises at least
twice a week.
Herbal teas like ginger tea can be enjoyed
before or after exercise to promote digestion,
reduce inflammation, and enhance recovery.

Medication:
Some individuals with diabetes may require
medication, such as insulin injections, oral
medications, or other injectable therapies, to
help manage blood sugar levels.
It's essential to take medications as prescribed
by healthcare providers and to monitor blood
sugar levels regularly to ensure optimal control.
Herbal teas, while not a replacement for
prescribed medications, can be incorporated
into a diabetes management plan to provide
additional support and potential benefits in
blood sugar control.

Complementary Approaches with Herbal Teas:

Herbal teas, such as fenugreek tea and holy basil tea, have been studied for their potential benefits in blood sugar control and may complement conventional diabetes management strategies.

Enjoying a cup of herbal tea as part of a balanced diet and lifestyle can provide hydration, relaxation, and potential health benefits without adding excess calories or sugar.

Experiment with different herbal tea recipes to find flavors and combinations that you enjoy, and consider incorporating them into your daily routine as a healthful and refreshing beverage option.

CHAPTER TWO

Benefits of Tea for Diabetes Management

Tea, one of the most consumed beverages worldwide, has garnered attention for its potential health benefits, particularly in diabetes management. From traditional herbal teas to classic green and black teas, incorporating tea into a diabetes management plan offers a flavorful and potentially beneficial way to support blood sugar control and overall well-being.

Antioxidant Properties:
Tea, particularly green tea, is rich in antioxidants known as polyphenols, which have been shown to have protective effects against oxidative stress and inflammation.

Antioxidants in tea may help reduce the risk of chronic diseases associated with diabetes, such as cardiovascular disease and diabetic complications.

Improved Insulin Sensitivity:
Some studies suggest that tea consumption, particularly green tea, may improve insulin sensitivity and enhance glucose metabolism. The polyphenols found in tea may help regulate insulin levels and support the body's ability to utilize glucose effectively, which is beneficial for individuals with diabetes.

Weight Management Support:
Tea, especially green tea, has been associated with modest reductions in body weight and body fat, which can be beneficial for individuals with diabetes, as excess weight can contribute to insulin resistance.
Drinking tea as part of a balanced diet and lifestyle may help support weight management efforts and improve metabolic health.

Cardiovascular Health Benefits:
Regular tea consumption has been linked to improvements in cardiovascular health, including reductions in blood pressure, cholesterol levels, and the risk of heart disease.
Individuals with diabetes are at increased risk of cardiovascular complications, making tea a valuable addition to a heart-healthy diet.

Hydration and Calorie-Free Beverage Option:
Tea is a calorie-free beverage option that can contribute to daily hydration needs without adding excess calories or sugar.
Choosing unsweetened tea over sugary beverages can help individuals with diabetes better manage their blood sugar levels and reduce the risk of weight gain and complications associated with excess sugar consumption.

Variety and Enjoyment:
With a wide variety of flavors and types available, tea offers endless opportunities for enjoyment and experimentation.
Herbal teas, such as cinnamon tea, ginger tea, and holy basil tea, provide unique flavors and potential health benefits that can complement a diabetes management plan.

The Science Behind Tea and Blood Sugar Regulation

Tea has long been revered for its health-promoting properties, and emerging research suggests that it may also play a role in blood sugar regulation, making it a potentially valuable addition to a diabetes management plan. Understanding the science behind how tea affects blood sugar levels can provide insights into its potential benefits and inform individuals with diabetes on how to incorporate tea into their daily routines.

Impact of Tea Polyphenols:
Tea contains a group of bioactive compounds known as polyphenols, which include catechins, theaflavins, and thearubigins. These polyphenols have antioxidant and anti-inflammatory properties that may contribute to their effects on blood sugar regulation.

Studies suggest that polyphenols in tea may improve insulin sensitivity, enhance glucose uptake by cells, and reduce insulin resistance, all of which are beneficial for individuals with diabetes.

Modulation of Glucose Metabolism:
Polyphenols found in tea, particularly catechins such as epigallocatechin gallate (EGCG) in green tea, may modulate glucose metabolism by inhibiting carbohydrate-digesting enzymes in the gut. This slows down the absorption of glucose into the bloodstream, resulting in more stable blood sugar levels after meals. Additionally, polyphenols may stimulate insulin secretion from pancreatic beta cells and enhance insulin action in peripheral tissues, further contributing to improved blood sugar control.

Antioxidant and Anti-Inflammatory Effects:
Oxidative stress and inflammation play key roles in the development and progression of diabetes and its complications. The antioxidant and anti-inflammatory properties of tea

polyphenols may help mitigate these factors and reduce the risk of diabetic complications. By neutralizing free radicals and suppressing inflammatory pathways, tea polyphenols may protect pancreatic beta cells from damage, improve endothelial function, and enhance insulin sensitivity.

Potential Benefits of Herbal Teas:
Herbal teas, made from various herbs and spices, also offer potential benefits in blood sugar regulation. For example, cinnamon contains compounds that mimic the effects of insulin and may help lower blood sugar levels. Ginger has been shown to improve insulin sensitivity and reduce fasting blood sugar levels, while fenugreek seeds may help slow down the absorption of sugar and improve insulin sensitivity.

Holy basil, another herb commonly used in herbal teas, may stimulate insulin secretion and help lower blood sugar levels, making it a valuable addition to diabetes management.

Considerations and Recommendations:
While tea and herbal teas offer potential benefits in blood sugar regulation, it's essential to consume them as part of a balanced diet and lifestyle.
Opt for unsweetened tea to avoid adding extra calories and sugar to your diet, and consider brewing your own herbal teas using natural ingredients for maximum health benefits. Individuals with diabetes should monitor their blood sugar levels regularly and consult with healthcare professionals before making significant changes to their diet or lifestyle, including the incorporation of tea into their routine.

The science behind tea and blood sugar regulation highlights the potential benefits of incorporating tea, particularly green tea and herbal teas, into a diabetes management plan. From its antioxidant and anti-inflammatory properties to its modulation of glucose metabolism, tea offers a natural and flavorful way to support blood sugar control and overall well-being. By understanding the mechanisms underlying tea's effects on blood sugar regulation, individuals with diabetes can make informed choices and enjoy the potential health benefits that tea has to offer.

Antioxidants and Polyphenols: Their Role in Diabetes Control

Antioxidants and polyphenols, found abundantly in certain foods and beverages like tea, play a crucial role in diabetes control. Understanding how these compounds work can provide valuable insights into their potential benefits for individuals managing diabetes. With the popularity of herbal teas on the rise, exploring the antioxidant and polyphenol content in these beverages offers a promising avenue for diabetes management.

Antioxidants:
Antioxidants are substances that prevent oxidative damage to cells and tissues in the body by neutralizing damaging free radicals. Oxidative stress is increased in diabetics, which can lead to issues like nerve damage and cardiovascular disease.

Antioxidants aid in lowering inflammation, enhancing insulin sensitivity, and preventing complications from diabetes by scavenging free radicals. Including foods and drinks high in antioxidants, like tea, in the diet can help manage diabetes and promote general health.

Polyphenols:
Polyphenols are a diverse group of phytochemicals found in plants, including fruits, vegetables, and tea. These compounds have attracted attention for their potential health benefits, including anti-inflammatory, antioxidant, and anti-diabetic properties. Within the category of polyphenols, flavonoids are of particular interest for their role in diabetes control. Flavonoids, such as catechins in green tea and quercetin in onions, berries, and apples, have been studied for their potential to improve insulin sensitivity and reduce blood sugar levels.

Role in Diabetes Control:
Antioxidants and polyphenols exert their effects on diabetes control through various mechanisms:

Improved Insulin Sensitivity: Polyphenols may enhance insulin sensitivity in peripheral tissues, allowing cells to better utilize glucose for energy.

Reduced Inflammation: Antioxidants and polyphenols possess anti-inflammatory properties that help mitigate chronic inflammation associated with insulin resistance and diabetic complications.

Protection of Beta Cells: Polyphenols may protect pancreatic beta cells from oxidative damage, preserving their function and insulin production capacity.

Enhanced Glucose Metabolism: Certain polyphenols, such as those found in tea, may modulate carbohydrate digestion and absorption, leading to more stable blood sugar levels after meals.

Incorporating Polyphenol-Rich Beverages:
Herbal teas, such as green tea, cinnamon tea, and ginger tea, are rich sources of polyphenols and antioxidants. Regular consumption of these beverages can contribute to overall polyphenol intake and support diabetes management.
Experimenting with different herbal tea recipes and incorporating a variety of antioxidant-rich foods into the diet can help individuals maximize their polyphenol intake and reap the potential health benefits associated with these compounds.

Considerations and Recommendations:
While antioxidants and polyphenols offer promising benefits for diabetes control, it's important to consume them as part of a balanced diet and lifestyle.
Individuals with diabetes should consult with healthcare professionals before making significant changes to their diet or incorporating new beverages, such as herbal teas, into their routine.

Monitoring blood sugar levels regularly and paying attention to overall dietary patterns can help individuals optimize their diabetes management efforts and support long-term health.

Antioxidants and polyphenols found in foods and beverages like herbal teas offer valuable support in diabetes control. By harnessing the power of these compounds, individuals with diabetes can take proactive steps to improve insulin sensitivity, reduce inflammation, and protect against diabetic complications. Incorporating antioxidant-rich herbal teas into a balanced diet offers a flavorful and healthful way to support overall well-being and enhance diabetes management efforts.

How Tea Consumption Can Support Overall Health in Diabetes

Tea consumption has been associated with numerous health benefits, including potential advantages for individuals managing diabetes. From improving insulin sensitivity to reducing inflammation and supporting heart health, incorporating tea into a diabetes management plan offers a holistic approach to overall well-being. Understanding how tea consumption can support various aspects of health in diabetes is essential for individuals looking to optimize their management strategies.

Improving Insulin Sensitivity:
Tea, particularly green tea, contains polyphenols such as catechins, which have been shown to improve insulin sensitivity in individuals with diabetes.

Enhanced insulin sensitivity allows cells to better respond to insulin, leading to improved glucose uptake and regulation.

Reducing Inflammation:
Chronic inflammation is a hallmark of diabetes and contributes to insulin resistance and complications such as cardiovascular disease. Tea polyphenols possess anti-inflammatory properties that help mitigate inflammation and reduce the risk of diabetic complications.

Supporting Heart Health:
Individuals with diabetes are at increased risk of heart disease, making cardiovascular health a priority in diabetes management. Tea consumption has been linked to improvements in cardiovascular health, including reductions in blood pressure, cholesterol levels, and the risk of heart disease.

Providing Hydration Without Added Sugars:
Choosing unsweetened tea as a beverage option provides hydration without the added sugars found in many other beverages. Staying hydrated is important for overall health and can help individuals with diabetes manage blood sugar levels more effectively.

Offering Variety and Enjoyment:
Tea comes in a wide variety of flavors and types, offering endless opportunities for enjoyment and experimentation. From classic green and black teas to herbal teas made from various herbs and spices, there's a tea to suit every taste preference.
Incorporating herbal teas, such as cinnamon tea, ginger tea, and holy basil tea, into a diabetes management plan adds variety to the diet while potentially offering additional health benefits.

Providing a Relaxing Ritual:
Enjoying a cup of tea can be a relaxing ritual that provides a moment of mindfulness and stress relief. Chronic stress can negatively impact blood sugar levels and overall health, so incorporating stress-reducing activities like tea drinking can be beneficial for individuals with diabetes.

Complementing a Balanced Diet and Lifestyle:
Tea consumption should be viewed as part of a balanced diet and lifestyle, alongside other healthy habits such as regular physical activity and mindful eating.
While tea can offer potential health benefits, it's important for individuals with diabetes to monitor their blood sugar levels regularly and consult with healthcare professionals to ensure that tea consumption fits into their overall diabetes management plan.

Incorporating tea consumption into a diabetes management plan offers numerous potential benefits for overall health. From improving insulin sensitivity and reducing inflammation to supporting heart health and providing hydration without added sugars, tea offers a flavorful and healthful addition to the diet. By enjoying a variety of teas as part of a balanced lifestyle, individuals with diabetes can take proactive steps to optimize their health and well-being while managing their condition effectively.

CHAPTER THREE

Herbal Tea Recipes for Lowering Blood Sugar

Herbal teas have long been valued for their potential health benefits, including their ability to help lower blood sugar levels. Incorporating herbal tea recipes into a diabetes management plan offers a natural and flavorful way to support blood sugar control. From cinnamon to fenugreek and beyond, these herbal tea recipes harness the power of nature's remedies to promote overall well-being in individuals with diabetes.

Cinnamon Tea:
Cinnamon is a popular spice known for its potential to help lower blood sugar levels by improving insulin sensitivity and slowing the absorption of glucose into the bloodstream.

To make cinnamon tea, steep a cinnamon stick
or cinnamon powder in hot water for 10-15
minutes. Optionally, add a squeeze of lemon or
a drizzle of honey for added flavor.

Ginger Tea:
Ginger contains compounds that may improve
insulin sensitivity and reduce fasting blood
sugar levels. Additionally, ginger has
anti-inflammatory properties that can benefit
individuals with diabetes.
To make ginger tea, thinly slice fresh ginger
root and steep it in hot water for 10-15 minutes.
For added flavor, you can also add a dash of
lemon juice or a sprinkle of cinnamon.

Fenugreek Tea:
Fenugreek seeds are rich in soluble fiber,
which can help slow down the absorption of
sugar and improve insulin sensitivity.
Fenugreek tea may also help reduce fasting
blood sugar levels.

To make fenugreek tea, steep fenugreek seeds in hot water for 10-15 minutes, then strain before drinking. You can adjust the strength of the tea by varying the amount of fenugreek seeds used.

Holy Basil Tea:
Holy basil, also known as tulsi, is revered in Ayurvedic medicine for its potential to help lower blood sugar levels by stimulating insulin secretion and improving glucose uptake.
To make holy basil tea, steep fresh or dried holy basil leaves in hot water for 5-10 minutes. You can enhance the flavor by adding a slice of lemon or a sprig of mint.

Green Tea with Cinnamon and Lemon:
Green tea contains catechins, antioxidants that may improve insulin sensitivity and reduce blood sugar levels. When combined with cinnamon and lemon, it creates a flavorful and healthful beverage for diabetes management.

To make green tea with cinnamon and lemon, steep a green tea bag in hot water for 2-3 minutes. Add a pinch of cinnamon powder and a squeeze of lemon juice before enjoying.

These herbal tea recipes offer a delightful and healthful way to support blood sugar control in individuals with diabetes. By incorporating ingredients like cinnamon, ginger, fenugreek, and holy basil into daily tea rituals, individuals can harness the power of nature's remedies to promote overall well-being and better manage their condition. Enjoying these herbal teas as part of a balanced diet and lifestyle can contribute to a holistic approach to diabetes management and improved quality of life.

Cinnamon Tea

Cinnamon tea is a delightful and healthful beverage that offers potential benefits for individuals managing diabetes. Cinnamon, a popular spice derived from the inner bark of the Cinnamomum tree, has been studied for its ability to help lower blood sugar levels and improve insulin sensitivity. Incorporating cinnamon tea into a diabetes management plan provides a flavorful and natural way to support blood sugar control and overall well-being.

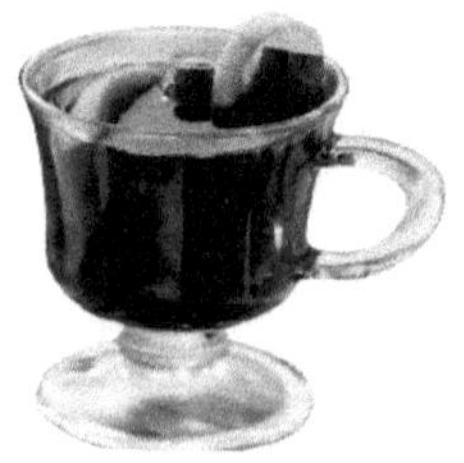

Health Benefits of Cinnamon:
Cinnamon contains bioactive compounds, such as cinnamaldehyde and cinnamic acid, which have antioxidant and anti-inflammatory properties.
Studies suggest that cinnamon may help improve insulin sensitivity, enhance glucose metabolism, and reduce fasting blood sugar levels, making it a valuable addition to a diabetes-friendly diet.

How to Make Cinnamon Tea:

Ingredients:
One teaspoon of ground cinnamon or one cinnamon stick
one cup of water
Guidelines:
In a small saucepan, bring the water to a rolling boil.
To the boiling water, add the ground cinnamon or cinnamon stick.
For ten to fifteen minutes, boil the cinnamon over low heat.

After turning off the heat, take the saucepan
and steep the cinnamon tea for five more
minutes.
To get rid of any remaining cinnamon, strain
the tea.
Warm up the cinnamon tea by pouring it into a
cup.

Variations of Cinnamon Tea:
Cinnamon Ginger Tea: Add a few slices of
fresh ginger root to the boiling water along with
the cinnamon for added flavor and potential
health benefits.
Cinnamon Lemon Tea: Squeeze a wedge of
lemon into the brewed cinnamon tea for a
refreshing citrus twist and extra vitamin C.
Cinnamon Honey Tea: Stir in a teaspoon of
honey into the brewed cinnamon tea for natural
sweetness and additional health benefits.

When to Enjoy Cinnamon Tea:
Cinnamon tea can be enjoyed at any time of the day as part of a balanced diet and lifestyle. Consider having a cup of cinnamon tea in the morning to kickstart your day or in the evening as a soothing and healthful beverage before bedtime.

Precautions and Considerations:
While cinnamon is generally safe for consumption, individuals taking medication for diabetes should consult with their healthcare provider before significantly increasing their cinnamon intake.
When incorporated into a broad and well-balanced diet, cinnamon tea should be consumed in moderation. Overindulgence could have negative effects such as an upset stomach.

Cinnamon tea offers a delicious and healthful way to incorporate the potential benefits of cinnamon into a diabetes management plan. Whether enjoyed plain or with added ingredients like ginger, lemon, or honey, cinnamon tea provides a flavorful and comforting beverage option for individuals looking to support blood sugar control and overall well-being. By incorporating cinnamon tea into their daily routines, individuals with diabetes can harness the power of this aromatic spice to enhance their quality of life and better manage their condition.

Ginger Tea

Ginger tea is a warming and aromatic beverage that offers potential benefits for individuals managing diabetes. Ginger, derived from the rhizome of the Zingiber plant, has been used for centuries in traditional medicine for its various health-promoting properties. Incorporating ginger tea into a diabetes management plan provides a flavorful and natural way to support blood sugar control and overall well-being.

Health Benefits of Ginger:
Ginger contains bioactive compounds, such as gingerol and shogaol, which have antioxidant and anti-inflammatory properties.
Studies suggest that ginger may help improve insulin sensitivity, reduce fasting blood sugar levels, and alleviate inflammation, making it a valuable addition to a diabetes-friendly diet.

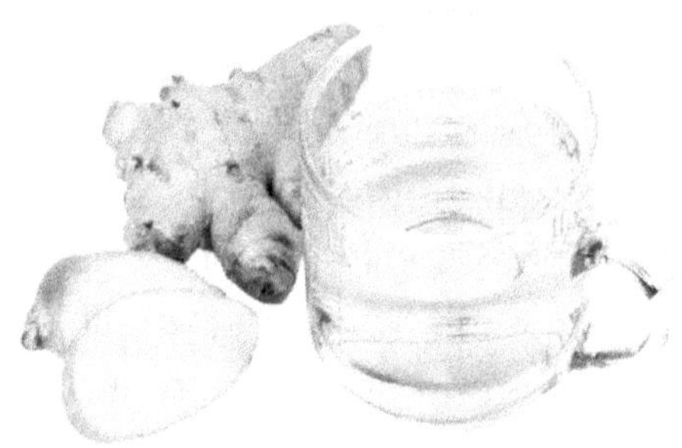

How to Make Ginger Tea:
Ingredients:
a finely sliced 1-inch piece of fresh ginger root
one cup of water
Guidelines:
In a small saucepan, bring the water to a rolling
boil.
Place the ginger root, finely sliced, into the
boiling water.

For ten to fifteen minutes, simmer the ginger over low heat.
After turning off the heat, take the saucepan and steep the ginger tea for five more minutes. To get rid of the ginger pieces, strain the tea. Warm up the ginger tea by pouring it into a cup.

Variations of Ginger Tea:
Ginger Lemon Tea: Squeeze a wedge of lemon into the brewed ginger tea for a refreshing citrus twist and extra vitamin C.
Ginger Honey Tea: Stir in a teaspoon of honey into the brewed ginger tea for natural sweetness and additional health benefits.
Ginger Turmeric Tea: Add a pinch of ground turmeric to the boiling water along with the ginger for added anti-inflammatory properties.

When to Enjoy Ginger Tea:
Ginger tea can be enjoyed at any time of the day as part of a balanced diet and lifestyle. Consider having a cup of ginger tea in the morning to invigorate your senses or in the evening as a soothing and healthful beverage before bedtime.

Warnings & Precautions: Although eating ginger is typically safe, people who are taking diabetes medication should speak with their doctor before consuming large amounts of ginger.
When consuming ginger tea as part of a varied and well-balanced diet, moderation is advised. Overindulgence could have negative effects such as an upset stomach.

Ginger tea offers a delightful and healthful way to incorporate the potential benefits of ginger into a diabetes management plan. Whether enjoyed plain or with added ingredients like lemon or honey, ginger tea provides a flavorful and comforting beverage option for individuals looking to support blood sugar control and overall well-being. By incorporating ginger tea into their daily routines, individuals with diabetes can harness the power of this aromatic root to enhance their quality of life and better manage their condition.

Fenugreek Tea

Fenugreek tea is a herbal beverage with a long history of use in traditional medicine for its potential health benefits, including its ability to help lower blood sugar levels. Fenugreek, derived from the seeds of the Trigonella foenum-graecum plant, contains soluble fiber and other bioactive compounds that may contribute to its effects on blood sugar regulation. Incorporating fenugreek tea into a diabetes management plan offers a flavorful and natural way to support blood sugar control and overall well-being.

Health Benefits of Fenugreek:
Fenugreek seeds are rich in soluble fiber, which can help slow down the absorption of sugar in the digestive tract and improve insulin sensitivity.

Studies suggest that fenugreek may help reduce fasting blood sugar levels, improve glucose tolerance, and enhance insulin action, making it a valuable addition to a diabetes-friendly diet.

How to Make Fenugreek Tea:

Ingredients:
1 teaspoon of fenugreek seeds
1 cup of water
Instructions:
Crush the fenugreek seeds slightly to release their flavor and aroma.
In a small saucepan, bring the water to a rolling boil.
Take the boiling water and add the crushed fenugreek seeds.
For ten to fifteen minutes, lower the heat and simmer the fenugreek.
After turning off the heat, take the pot off the burner and steep the fenugreek tea for five more minutes.

To get rid of the fenugreek seeds, strain the tea.
Warm up the fenugreek tea by pouring it into a cup.

Variations of Fenugreek Tea:

Fenugreek Cinnamon Tea: Add a cinnamon stick or a pinch of ground cinnamon to the boiling water along with the fenugreek seeds for added flavor and potential health benefits.
Fenugreek Lemon Tea: Squeeze a wedge of lemon into the brewed fenugreek tea for a refreshing citrus twist and extra vitamin C.
Fenugreek Honey Tea: Stir in a teaspoon of honey into the brewed fenugreek tea for natural sweetness and additional health benefits.

When to Enjoy Fenugreek Tea:
Fenugreek tea can be enjoyed at any time of
the day as part of a balanced diet and lifestyle.
Consider having a cup of fenugreek tea before
meals to help improve glucose tolerance and
support blood sugar control.

Precautions and Considerations:
Although fenugreek is typically safe to eat,
before drastically increasing their fenugreek
intake, people on diabetes medication should
speak with their healthcare professional.
When incorporated into a broad and
well-balanced diet, fenugreek tea should be
used in moderation. Overindulgence could
have negative effects such as an upset
stomach.

Fenugreek tea offers a flavorful and healthful
way to incorporate the potential benefits of
fenugreek into a diabetes management plan.
Whether enjoyed plain or with added
ingredients like cinnamon, lemon, or honey,

fenugreek tea provides a comforting and beneficial beverage option for individuals looking to support blood sugar control and overall well-being. By incorporating fenugreek tea into their daily routines, individuals with diabetes can harness the power of this ancient herb to enhance their quality of life and better manage their condition.

Turmeric Tea

Turmeric tea, also known as golden milk or turmeric latte, is a popular beverage with origins in traditional Ayurvedic medicine. Turmeric, a bright yellow spice derived from the Curcuma longa plant, contains a compound called curcumin, which has been studied for its potential health benefits, including its effects on blood sugar regulation. Incorporating turmeric tea into a diabetes management plan offers a flavorful and natural way to support blood sugar control and overall well-being.

Health Benefits of Turmeric:
Turmeric's main ingredient, curcumin, has strong anti-inflammatory and antioxidant qualities.
Turmeric is a great addition to a diabetes-friendly diet since studies suggest that curcumin may help enhance insulin sensitivity, reduce inflammation, and lower fasting blood sugar levels.

How to Make Turmeric Tea:

Ingredients:
1 tablespoon of freshly grated turmeric root or
1 teaspoon of crushed turmeric
One cup of milk, either plant-based or dairy
One teaspoon of optional maple syrup or
honey
A small amount of black pepper (which
improves curcumin absorption)

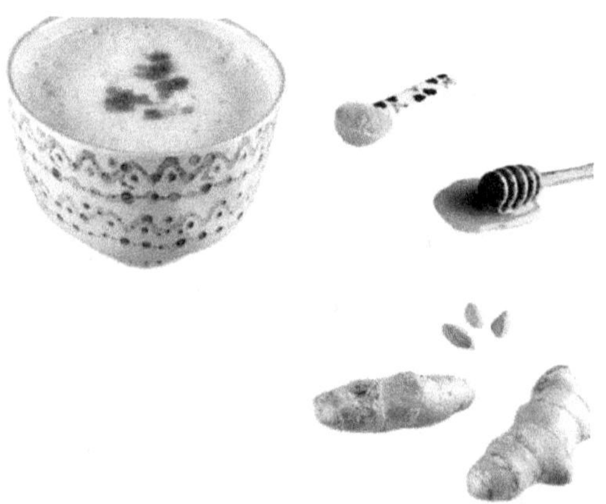

Instructions:
In a small saucepan, heat the milk over medium heat until warm but not boiling.
Add the ground turmeric or grated fresh turmeric root to the warm milk.
Stir in the honey or maple syrup if desired, and add a pinch of black pepper.
Continue to heat the turmeric milk mixture for 3-5 minutes, stirring occasionally.
Remove the saucepan from the heat and strain the turmeric tea into a cup.
Enjoy hot as a comforting and healthful beverage.

Variations of Turmeric Tea:
Turmeric Ginger Tea: Add a few slices of fresh ginger root to the turmeric milk mixture for added flavor and potential health benefits.
Turmeric Cinnamon Tea: Sprinkle a pinch of ground cinnamon into the turmeric milk mixture for a warm and spicy flavor profile.
Turmeric Cardamom Tea: Add a dash of ground cardamom to the turmeric milk mixture for a fragrant and exotic twist.

When to Enjoy Turmeric Tea:
Turmeric tea can be enjoyed at any time of the
day as part of a balanced diet and lifestyle.
Consider having a cup of turmeric tea in the
morning to kickstart your day or in the evening
as a soothing and healthful beverage before
bedtime.

Warnings and Recommendations: Although
consuming turmeric is typically safe, people
who are taking diabetes medication should
speak with their doctor before drastically
increasing their use of turmeric.
Consuming turmeric tea in moderation as a
component of a diverse and well-rounded diet
is recommended. Overindulgence could have
negative effects such as an upset stomach.

Turmeric tea offers a delicious and healthful
way to incorporate the potential benefits of
turmeric into a diabetes management plan.
Whether enjoyed plain or with added
ingredients like ginger, cinnamon, or

cardamom, turmeric tea provides a flavorful and comforting beverage option for individuals looking to support blood sugar control and overall well-being. By incorporating turmeric tea into their daily routines, individuals with diabetes can harness the power of this vibrant spice to enhance their quality of life and better manage their condition.

Bitter Melon Tea

Bitter melon, also known as bitter gourd or Momordica charantia, is a tropical vine widely cultivated for its edible fruit, which has a distinctively bitter taste. Bitter melon has been used in traditional medicine for centuries, particularly in Asian and African cultures, for its potential health benefits, including its effects on blood sugar regulation. Incorporating bitter melon tea into a diabetes management plan offers a flavorful and natural way to support blood sugar control and overall well-being.

Health Benefits of Bitter Melon:
Bitter melon contains bioactive compounds, including charantin, vicine, and polypeptide-p, which have been studied for their potential antidiabetic properties.
Studies suggest that bitter melon may help lower blood sugar levels, improve insulin sensitivity, and reduce the risk of diabetic complications, making it a valuable addition to a diabetes-friendly diet.

How to Make Bitter Melon Tea:

Ingredients:
1 bitter melon, sliced (seeds removed)
2 cups of water
Instructions:
In a small saucepan, bring the water to a rolling
boil.
Pour the boiling water over the cut bitter melon.
For ten to fifteen minutes, boil the bitter melon
over low heat.
After turning off the heat, take the saucepan
and steep the bitter melon tea for five more
minutes.
Remove the bitter melon slices from the tea by
straining it.
Transfer the acrid melon tea into a cup and
relish it warm.

Variations of Bitter Melon Tea:
Bitter Melon Lemon Tea: Squeeze a wedge of
lemon into the brewed bitter melon tea for a
refreshing citrus twist and extra vitamin C.

Bitter Melon Mint Tea: Add a few fresh mint leaves to the boiling water along with the bitter melon for a cool and refreshing flavor.

When to Enjoy Bitter Melon Tea:
Bitter melon tea can be enjoyed at any time of the day as part of a balanced diet and lifestyle. Consider having a cup of bitter melon tea before meals to help improve glucose tolerance and support blood sugar control.

Precautions and Considerations:
Bitter melon tea may not be suitable for everyone, as some individuals may find its taste too bitter.
Individuals taking medication for diabetes should consult with their healthcare provider before significantly increasing their bitter melon intake, as it may interact with certain medications or affect blood sugar levels.

Bitter melon tea offers a unique and healthful way to incorporate the potential benefits of bitter melon into a diabetes management plan. Whether enjoyed plain or with added ingredients like lemon or mint, bitter melon tea provides a flavorful and beneficial beverage option for individuals looking to support blood sugar control and overall well-being. By incorporating bitter melon tea into their daily routines, individuals with diabetes can explore the potential of this tropical fruit to enhance their quality of life and better manage their condition.

CHAPTER FOUR

Green Tea Infusions for Diabetes Control

Green tea, renowned for its numerous health benefits, has gained popularity for its potential role in diabetes control. Rich in antioxidants and bioactive compounds, green tea offers a flavorful and natural way to support blood sugar regulation and overall well-being. By exploring different green tea infusions, individuals managing diabetes can enhance their diabetes management plan and enjoy a variety of delicious beverages.

Health Benefits of Green Tea:
Green tea contains polyphenols, particularly catechins like epigallocatechin gallate (EGCG), which have antioxidant and anti-inflammatory properties.

Studies suggest that green tea may help improve insulin sensitivity, reduce fasting blood sugar levels, and mitigate oxidative stress, making it beneficial for individuals with diabetes.

Basic Green Tea Infusion:

Ingredients:
1 teaspoon of green tea leaves or 1 green tea bag
1 cup of hot water

Instructions:
Put the bag or leaves of green tea into a cup.
Cover the tea leaves or bag with hot water.
Steep for a moderate brew for two to three minutes, or up to five minutes for a stronger flavor.
Take out the tea leaves or bag and savor your brew of green tea.

Variations of Green Tea Infusions:

Green Tea with Lemon: Add a slice of fresh lemon to your green tea infusion for a refreshing citrus twist and added vitamin C.
Green Tea with Mint: Add a few fresh mint leaves to your green tea infusion for a cool and invigorating flavor.
Green Tea with Cinnamon: Sprinkle a pinch of ground cinnamon into your green tea infusion for a warm and spicy flavor profile that may help further support blood sugar control.

Matcha Green Tea Latte:
Matcha powder is a concentrated form of green tea that offers even higher levels of antioxidants and beneficial compounds.

Ingredients:
Matcha powder, one teaspoon
One cup of heated milk (vegan or dairy)
Sweeteners of choice (such as honey or maple syrup) are optional.

Guidelines:
Mix the matcha powder and a tiny bit of boiling water in a cup to make a paste.
The milk should be warmed but not boiling.
After adding the heated milk to the matcha paste, thoroughly mix everything together.
If preferred, sweeten to taste.
Savor the rich, delicious, and creamy matcha green tea latte.

Incorporating Green Tea Infusions into Daily Routine:
Green tea infusions can be enjoyed throughout the day as part of a balanced diet and lifestyle. Consider having a cup of green tea with meals or as a mid-morning or afternoon pick-me-up.

Precautions and Considerations:
While green tea is generally safe for consumption, individuals sensitive to caffeine should monitor their intake, as green tea contains caffeine.

Individuals taking medication for diabetes should consult with their healthcare provider before significantly increasing their green tea consumption, as it may interact with certain medications or affect blood sugar levels.

Green tea infusions offer a flavorful and healthful way to incorporate the potential benefits of green tea into a diabetes management plan. Whether enjoyed plain or with added ingredients like lemon, mint, or cinnamon, green tea infusions provide a delicious and beneficial beverage option for individuals looking to support blood sugar control and overall well-being. By incorporating green tea infusions into their daily routines, individuals with diabetes can explore the potential of this ancient beverage to enhance their quality of life and better manage their condition.

Green Tea and EGCG: Impact on Insulin Sensitivity

Green tea, revered for its health-promoting properties, contains high levels of antioxidants and bioactive compounds, including epigallocatechin gallate (EGCG). EGCG, a catechin found abundantly in green tea, has garnered attention for its potential impact on insulin sensitivity and blood sugar regulation. Understanding the role of green tea and EGCG in improving insulin sensitivity is crucial for individuals managing diabetes.

Understanding Insulin Sensitivity:
Insulin sensitivity refers to how effectively the body's cells respond to insulin, the hormone responsible for regulating blood sugar levels. Reduced insulin sensitivity, known as insulin resistance, is a key factor in the development of type 2 diabetes and can lead to elevated blood sugar levels and metabolic disturbances.

Impact of Green Tea and EGCG on Insulin Sensitivity:

Studies suggest that EGCG, the primary polyphenol in green tea, may help improve insulin sensitivity through various mechanisms: Enhanced Glucose Uptake: EGCG may increase glucose uptake in skeletal muscle cells, enhancing their ability to utilize glucose for energy.

Activation of AMPK: EGCG has been shown to activate adenosine monophosphate-activated protein kinase (AMPK), an enzyme involved in cellular energy metabolism and insulin sensitivity.

Reduced Inflammation: EGCG possesses anti-inflammatory properties that may help mitigate chronic inflammation associated with insulin resistance.

Protection Against Beta Cell Dysfunction: EGCG may protect pancreatic beta cells from oxidative stress and apoptosis, preserving their function and insulin secretion capacity.

Clinical Evidence Supporting EGCG's Effects:

Clinical trials have demonstrated the potential benefits of green tea and EGCG supplementation on insulin sensitivity and

blood sugar control:

A study published in the Journal of Agricultural and Food Chemistry found that green tea consumption improved insulin sensitivity and reduced fasting blood sugar levels in individuals with type 2 diabetes.

Another study published in The American Journal of Clinical Nutrition reported that EGCG supplementation improved insulin sensitivity and reduced markers of inflammation in overweight and obese individuals.

Including Green Tea in a Diabetes Treatment Strategy:

Drinking green tea can help boost insulin sensitivity and blood sugar control in a tasty and beneficial way when used as part of a balanced diet and lifestyle.

Make sure you have two to three cups of green tea every day to get the possible health advantages of EGCG and other bioactive ingredients.

Precautions and Considerations:

While green tea is generally safe for consumption, individuals sensitive to caffeine should monitor their intake, as green tea contains caffeine.

Individuals taking medication for diabetes should consult with their healthcare provider before significantly increasing their green tea consumption, as it may interact with certain medications or affect blood sugar levels.

Green tea, rich in EGCG and other antioxidants, offers a promising avenue for improving insulin sensitivity and supporting blood sugar control in individuals managing diabetes. By incorporating green tea into their daily routines as part of a balanced diet and lifestyle, individuals can harness the potential benefits of EGCG to enhance their diabetes management efforts and improve overall well-being. Enjoying green tea as a flavorful beverage option can be a simple yet effective strategy for supporting insulin sensitivity and optimizing blood sugar regulation in individuals with diabetes.

Matcha Green Tea

Matcha green tea, a powdered form of green tea made from finely ground tea leaves, has gained popularity for its unique flavor and potential health benefits. Rich in antioxidants, including catechins like epigallocatechin gallate (EGCG), matcha offers a flavorful and healthful beverage option for individuals managing diabetes. Understanding the potential impact of matcha green tea on blood sugar regulation and overall well-being is essential for incorporating it into a diabetes management plan.

Health Benefits of Matcha Green Tea:
Matcha contains high levels of antioxidants, particularly EGCG, which have been studied for their potential health-promoting properties. The concentrated form of matcha powder allows for a higher intake of antioxidants compared to traditional steeped green tea, potentially enhancing its benefits.

Impact on Blood Sugar Regulation:
Research indicates that the antioxidants in matcha green tea, especially EGCG, may help control blood sugar levels and enhance insulin sensitivity.
Increased insulin sensitivity can help the body use glucose more efficiently, which lowers the chance of high blood sugar and insulin resistance.

How to Prepare Matcha Green Tea:

Ingredients:
1 teaspoon of matcha green tea powder
Hot water (not boiling)
Optional: sweetener of choice (e.g., honey, maple syrup)

Instructions:
If there are any clumps, sift the matcha powder into a bowl.
Bring the water's temperature down to about 175°F (80°C), but not quite boiling.
Add a tiny amount of hot water to the matcha powder-filled bowl.
Blend the matcha and water until frothy and smooth with a bamboo whisk or an electric frother.
Add the remaining hot water little by little while whisking until thoroughly blended.
If preferred, sweeten to taste.
Enjoy the matcha green tea after pouring it into a cup.

Variations of Matcha Green Tea:

Matcha Latte: Replace some or all of the hot water with hot milk (dairy or plant-based) for a creamy and indulgent matcha latte.

Matcha Smoothie: Blend matcha powder with fruits, vegetables, and your choice of milk or yogurt to create a nutritious and energizing matcha smoothie.

Incorporating Matcha Green Tea into a Diabetes Management Plan:
Enjoying matcha green tea as part of a balanced diet and lifestyle can provide a flavorful and healthful way to support blood sugar control and overall well-being.
Aim to consume matcha green tea regularly, but be mindful of added sweeteners if managing carbohydrate intake.

Precautions and Considerations:
While matcha green tea is generally safe for consumption, individuals sensitive to caffeine should monitor their intake, as matcha contains caffeine.

Individuals taking medication for diabetes should consult with their healthcare provider before significantly increasing their matcha consumption, as it may interact with certain medications or affect blood sugar levels.

Matcha green tea offers a delicious and healthful beverage option for individuals managing diabetes. Rich in antioxidants like EGCG, matcha green tea may help improve insulin sensitivity and support blood sugar regulation when incorporated into a diabetes management plan. By enjoying matcha green tea as part of a balanced diet and lifestyle, individuals can harness its potential benefits to enhance their overall well-being and better manage their condition.

Sencha Green Tea

Sencha green tea, a staple in Japanese tea culture, is renowned for its refreshing flavor and potential health benefits. Made from the first tender leaves of the Camellia plant, sencha green tea is rich in antioxidants, particularly catechins like epigallocatechin gallate (EGCG). Incorporating sencha green tea into a diabetes management plan offers a flavorful and natural way to support blood sugar control and overall well-being.

Health Benefits of Sencha Green Tea:
Sencha green tea contains high levels of antioxidants, including EGCG, which have been studied for their potential health-promoting properties.
The unique cultivation and processing methods of sencha green tea result in a vibrant flavor profile and a higher concentration of beneficial compounds compared to other green teas.

Impact on Blood Sugar Regulation:
Studies suggest that the antioxidants found in sencha green tea, particularly EGCG, may help improve insulin sensitivity and regulate blood sugar levels.
Enhanced insulin sensitivity can lead to better glucose uptake by cells, reducing the risk of elevated blood sugar levels and insulin resistance.

How to Prepare Sencha Green Tea:

Ingredients:
1 teaspoon of sencha green tea leaves or 1 sencha green tea bag
Hot water (not boiling).

Instructions:
Place the sencha green tea leaves or bag in a cup or teapot.
Heat the water to approximately 175°F (80°C), just below boiling.

Pour the hot water over the sencha green tea leaves or bag.

Steep for 1-2 minutes for a mild flavor or up to 3 minutes for a stronger brew.

Remove the tea leaves or bag and enjoy your sencha green tea.

Variations of Sencha Green Tea:

Sencha Lemon Tea: Add a slice of fresh lemon to your sencha green tea for a refreshing citrus twist and added vitamin C.

Sencha Mint Tea: Add a few fresh mint leaves to your sencha green tea for a cool and invigorating flavor.

Incorporating Sencha Green Tea into a Diabetes Management Plan:

Enjoying sencha green tea as part of a balanced diet and lifestyle can provide a flavorful and healthful way to support blood sugar control and overall well-being.

Aim to drink 2-3 cups of sencha green tea per day to reap the potential benefits of its antioxidants and other bioactive compounds.

Precautions and Considerations:
Sencha green tea is generally safe for consumption, but individuals sensitive to caffeine should monitor their intake, as sencha contains caffeine.
Individuals taking medication for diabetes should consult with their healthcare provider before significantly increasing their sencha green tea consumption, as it may interact with certain medications or affect blood sugar levels.

Sencha green tea offers a delightful and healthful beverage option for individuals managing diabetes. With its rich antioxidant content, particularly EGCG, sencha green tea may help improve insulin sensitivity and support blood sugar regulation when incorporated into a diabetes management plan. By enjoying sencha green tea as part of a balanced diet and lifestyle, individuals can harness its potential benefits to enhance their overall well-being and better manage their condition.

Jasmine Green Tea

Jasmine green tea is a fragrant and flavorful beverage that combines the health benefits of green tea with the delicate aroma of jasmine flowers. Made by infusing green tea leaves with jasmine blossoms, this tea offers a refreshing and soothing drink that can be enjoyed throughout the day. Incorporating jasmine green tea into a diabetes management plan provides a delicious and natural way to support blood sugar control and overall well-being.

Health Benefits of Jasmine Green Tea:
Jasmine green tea contains the antioxidants and polyphenols found in green tea, including catechins like epigallocatechin gallate (EGCG), which have been studied for their potential health-promoting properties.
The addition of jasmine flowers provides aromatic compounds that may offer additional health benefits, including relaxation and stress relief.

Impact on Blood Sugar Regulation:
Studies suggest that the antioxidants found in green tea, such as EGCG, may help improve insulin sensitivity and regulate blood sugar levels.

By supporting insulin sensitivity, jasmine green tea can aid in glucose uptake by cells, potentially reducing the risk of elevated blood sugar levels and insulin resistance.

How to Prepare Jasmine Green Tea:

Ingredients:
1 teaspoon of jasmine green tea leaves or 1 jasmine green tea bag
Hot water (not boiling).

Instructions:
Place the jasmine green tea leaves or bag in a cup or teapot.
Heat the water to approximately 175°F (80°C), just below boiling.

Pour the hot water over the jasmine green tea leaves or bag.
Steep for 2-3 minutes to allow the flavors to infuse.
Remove the tea leaves or bag and enjoy your fragrant jasmine green tea.

Variations of Jasmine Green Tea:
Jasmine Green Tea with Lemon: Add a slice of fresh lemon to your jasmine green tea for a zesty twist and an extra boost of vitamin C.
Jasmine Green Tea with Honey: Stir in a teaspoon of honey to your jasmine green tea for natural sweetness and added flavor.

Incorporating Jasmine Green Tea into a Diabetes Management Plan:
Enjoying jasmine green tea as part of a balanced diet and lifestyle can provide a delicious and healthful way to support blood sugar control and overall well-being.
Aim to include jasmine green tea as a regular beverage option, alongside other diabetes-friendly choices.

Precautions and Considerations:
Jasmine green tea is generally safe for
consumption, but individuals sensitive to
caffeine should monitor their intake, as green
tea contains caffeine.
Individuals taking medication for diabetes
should consult with their healthcare provider
before significantly increasing their jasmine
green tea consumption, as it may interact with
certain medications or affect blood sugar
levels.

Jasmine green tea offers a delightful and
aromatic beverage option for individuals
managing diabetes. With its blend of green tea
antioxidants and jasmine floral notes, jasmine
green tea provides a flavorful and healthful
addition to a diabetes management plan. By
incorporating jasmine green tea into their daily
routines, individuals can enjoy its potential
benefits for blood sugar control and overall
well-being, all while savoring its soothing
aroma and refreshing taste.

Moroccan Mint Green Tea

Moroccan mint green tea, also known as " bi nana," is a traditional beverage enjoyed throughout Morocco and other parts of North Africa. This refreshing tea combines the health benefits of green tea with the cooling and invigorating flavor of fresh mint leaves. Incorporating Moroccan mint green tea into a diabetes management plan offers a delicious and natural way to support blood sugar control and overall well-being.

Health Benefits of Moroccan Mint Green Tea:

Moroccan mint green tea contains the antioxidants and polyphenols found in green tea, including catechins like epigallocatechin gallate (EGCG), which have been studied for their potential health-promoting properties. The addition of fresh mint leaves provides additional health benefits, including digestive support, relaxation, and a cooling sensation.

Impact on Blood Sugar Regulation:
Studies suggest that the antioxidants found in green tea, such as EGCG, may help improve insulin sensitivity and regulate blood sugar levels.
By supporting insulin sensitivity, Moroccan mint green tea can aid in glucose uptake by cells, potentially reducing the risk of elevated blood sugar levels and insulin resistance.

How to Prepare Moroccan Mint Green Tea:

Ingredients:
1 teaspoon of green tea leaves or 1 green tea bag
A handful of fresh mint leaves
Hot water (not boiling)
Instructions:
Place the green tea leaves or bag in a teapot or heat proof pitcher.
Add the fresh mint leaves to the teapot.
Heat the water to approximately 175°F (80°C), just below boiling.

Pour the hot water over the green tea leaves and mint leaves.
Steep for 2-3 minutes to allow the flavors to infuse.
Strain the tea to remove the tea leaves and mint leaves.
Pour the Moroccan mint green tea into cups and enjoy.

Variations of Moroccan Mint Green Tea:

Moroccan Mint Green Tea with Lemon: Add a slice of fresh lemon to your tea for a citrusy twist and an extra burst of flavor.
Moroccan Mint Green Tea with Honey: Stir in a teaspoon of honey to your tea for natural sweetness and added depth of flavor.

Incorporating Moroccan Mint Green Tea into a Diabetes Management Plan:
Enjoying Moroccan mint green tea as part of a balanced diet and lifestyle can provide a flavorful and healthful way to support blood sugar control and overall well-being.

Aim to include Moroccan mint green tea as a regular beverage option, alongside other diabetes-friendly choices.

Precautions and Considerations:
Moroccan mint green tea is generally safe for consumption, but individuals sensitive to caffeine should monitor their intake, as green tea contains caffeine.
Individuals taking medication for diabetes should consult with their healthcare provider before significantly increasing their Moroccan mint green tea consumption, as it may interact with certain medications or affect blood sugar levels.

Moroccan mint green tea offers a refreshing and aromatic beverage option for individuals managing diabetes. With its blend of green tea antioxidants and fresh mint leaves, Moroccan mint green tea provides a flavorful and healthful addition to a diabetes management plan. By incorporating Moroccan mint green tea into their daily routines, individuals can enjoy its potential benefits for blood sugar control and overall well-being, all while savoring its cooling sensation and invigorating taste.

CHAPTER FIVE

Spice-infused Tea Blends for Managing Diabetes

Spice-infused tea blends offer a delightful and flavorful way to support blood sugar management and overall well-being for individuals with diabetes. By combining various spices with tea leaves, these aromatic blends provide a delicious alternative to traditional beverages while harnessing the potential health benefits of spices. Incorporating spice-infused tea blends into a diabetes management plan can add variety to the diet and contribute to improved blood sugar control.

Health Benefits of Spice-Infused Tea Blends:

Spices like cinnamon, ginger, turmeric, and fenugreek are known for their potential to improve insulin sensitivity, regulate blood sugar levels, and reduce inflammation.

Combining these spices with tea leaves enhances their bioavailability and makes them easier to incorporate into daily routines.

Popular Spice-Infused Tea Blends for Managing Diabetes:

1. **Cinnamon Tea:** Cinnamon has been studied for its ability to lower fasting blood sugar levels and improve insulin sensitivity. Brewing cinnamon tea by steeping cinnamon sticks or ground cinnamon in hot water provides a warm and comforting beverage option.

2. **Ginger Tea**: Ginger contains gingerol, a compound known for its anti-inflammatory and antioxidant properties. Ginger tea can help improve digestion, reduce nausea, and potentially lower blood sugar levels when consumed regularly.

3. **Turmeric Tea**: Turmeric contains curcumin, a potent antioxidant with anti-inflammatory properties. Turmeric tea offers a vibrant and earthy flavor while providing potential benefits for blood sugar control and overall health.

4. **Fenugreek Tea**: Fenugreek seeds are rich in soluble fiber and compounds that may help improve insulin sensitivity and regulate blood sugar levels. Brewing fenugreek tea by steeping fenugreek seeds in hot water offers a slightly bitter yet healthful beverage option.

How to Prepare Spice-Infused Tea Blends:

Ingredients:
Tea leaves (green tea, black tea, or herbal tea)
Spices of choice (cinnamon sticks, ginger slices, turmeric powder, fenugreek seeds)
Hot water.

Instructions:
Choose your desired tea leaves and spices based on flavor preferences and health goals.
Add the tea leaves and spices to a teapot or heat proof pitcher.
Cover the tea leaves and spices with hot water.
Depending on the intensity that you want, let the blend steep for five to ten minutes.
To get rid of the spices and tea leaves, strain the tea.
Warm up the tea with added spices and savor it.

Incorporating Spice-Infused Tea Blends into a Diabetes Management Plan:
Enjoying spice-infused tea blends as part of a balanced diet and lifestyle can provide a flavorful and healthful way to support blood sugar control and overall well-being.
Experiment with different spice combinations and tea bases to find your favorite blends and incorporate them into your daily routine.

Precautions and Considerations:
While spices are generally safe for consumption, individuals with certain medical conditions or allergies should consult with a healthcare provider before incorporating spice-infused tea blends into their diet. Monitor blood sugar levels regularly and adjust consumption as needed based on individual response.

Spice-infused tea blends offer a delicious and healthful option for individuals managing diabetes. By combining tea leaves with spices like cinnamon, ginger, turmeric, and fenugreek, these blends provide a flavorful way to support blood sugar management and overall well-being. Incorporating spice-infused tea blends into a diabetes management plan can add variety to the diet and contribute to improved blood sugar control, all while enjoying the aromatic and comforting flavors of spices

Chai Tea

Chai tea, a spiced tea originating from India, has become a beloved beverage around the world for its rich flavor and aromatic spices. Traditionally made with black tea, milk, and a blend of spices like cinnamon, cardamom, ginger, and cloves, chai tea offers a comforting and invigorating experience. Incorporating chai tea into a diabetes management plan provides a flavorful and healthful way to enjoy the benefits of spices while supporting blood sugar control and overall well-being.

Health Benefits of Chai Tea:
Chai tea contains a variety of spices, each offering potential health benefits. Cinnamon, for example, has been studied for its ability to improve insulin sensitivity and regulate blood sugar levels.
Black tea, the base of chai tea, is rich in antioxidants called flavonoids, which may have protective effects against chronic diseases.

Impact on Blood Sugar Regulation:
The spices commonly found in chai tea, such as cinnamon and ginger, have been studied for their potential to improve insulin sensitivity and regulate blood sugar levels.
By incorporating chai tea into a diabetes management plan, individuals may benefit from the potential blood sugar-lowering effects of these spices.

How to Prepare Chai Tea:
Ingredients:
1 cup of water
1 black tea bag or 1 tablespoon of loose black tea leaves
1/2 cup of milk (dairy or plant-based)
Spices: cinnamon sticks, cardamom pods, cloves, ginger slices
Sweetener of choice (optional).

Instructions:
Heat the water in a small saucepan until it boils.
Add the black tea bag or tea leaves to the boiling water.
Add the spices to the saucepan, adjusting the quantities to suit your taste preferences.
Simmer the tea and spices for 3-5 minutes to allow the flavors to infuse.
Add the milk to the saucepan and continue to simmer for an additional 2-3 minutes.
Remove the saucepan from the heat and let the chai tea steep for a few minutes.
Strain the chai tea into cups, add sweetener if desired, and enjoy.

Variations of Chai Tea:

Decaffeinated Chai Tea: Use decaffeinated black tea to reduce caffeine intake, especially for those sensitive to caffeine.
Spiced Chai Latte: Froth the milk before adding it to the chai tea for a creamy and indulgent beverage.

Incorporating Chai Tea into a Diabetes Management Plan:

Enjoying chai tea as part of a balanced diet and lifestyle can provide a flavorful and healthful way to support blood sugar control and overall well-being.
Be mindful of added sweeteners, especially for individuals managing carbohydrate intake.

Precautions and Considerations:

Individuals with lactose intolerance or dairy allergies can use plant-based milk alternatives like almond, soy, or coconut milk.
Monitor blood sugar levels regularly and adjust chai tea consumption as needed based on individual response.

Chai tea offers a delicious and aromatic beverage option for individuals managing diabetes. With its blend of spices and black tea, chai tea provides a flavorful and healthful addition to a diabetes management plan. By incorporating chai tea into their daily routines, individuals can enjoy its potential benefits for blood sugar control and overall well-being, all while savoring it's comforting and invigorating flavors.

Cardamom Tea

Cardamom tea, also known as elaichi chai, is a fragrant and flavorful beverage that combines the warmth of black tea with the distinct aroma of cardamom pods. Originating from South Asia, cardamom tea is cherished for its aromatic properties and potential health benefits. Incorporating cardamom tea into a diabetes management plan offers a delicious and natural way to support blood sugar control and overall well-being.

Health Benefits of Cardamom Tea:
Cardamom is rich in antioxidants and essential oils, which contribute to its potential health-promoting properties.
Studies suggest that cardamom may help improve digestion, reduce inflammation, and regulate blood sugar levels, making it beneficial for individuals managing diabetes.

Impact on Blood Sugar Regulation:
The antioxidants found in cardamom, such as polyphenols and flavonoids, may help improve insulin sensitivity and regulate blood sugar levels.
By incorporating cardamom tea into a diabetes management plan, individuals may benefit from the potential blood sugar-lowering effects of this aromatic spice.

How to Prepare Cardamom Tea:

Ingredients:
1 cup of water
1 black tea bag or 1 tablespoon of loose black tea leaves
2-3 cardamom pods, crushed or lightly crushed
Sweetener of choice (optional).

Instructions:
In a small saucepan, bring the water to a boil.
Add the black tea bag or tea leaves to the boiling water.

Add the crushed cardamom pods to the saucepan.
Simmer the tea and cardamom for 3-5 minutes to allow the flavors to infuse.
Remove the saucepan from the heat and let the tea steep for a few minutes.
Strain the cardamom tea into cups, add sweetener if desired, and enjoy.

Variations of Cardamom Tea:
Creamy Cardamom Tea: Add a splash of milk (dairy or plant-based) to the tea for a creamy and indulgent beverage.
Cardamom Green Tea: Substitute black tea with green tea for a lighter and more delicate flavor profile.

Incorporating Cardamom Tea into a Diabetes Management Plan:
Enjoying cardamom tea as part of a balanced diet and lifestyle can provide a flavorful and healthful way to support blood sugar control and overall well-being.
Be mindful of added sweeteners, especially for individuals managing carbohydrate intake.

Precautions and Considerations:
Individuals with gastrointestinal issues or sensitivities to spices should consume cardamom tea in moderation.
Monitor blood sugar levels regularly and adjust cardamom tea consumption as needed based on individual response.

Cardamom tea offers a fragrant and aromatic beverage option for individuals managing diabetes. With its blend of black tea and cardamom pods, cardamom tea provides a flavorful and healthful addition to a diabetes management plan. By incorporating cardamom tea into their daily routines, individuals can enjoy its potential benefits for blood sugar control and overall well-being, all while savoring its aromatic and comforting flavors.

Clove Tea

Clove tea is a fragrant and flavorful beverage made from dried cloves, the flower buds of the clove tree. Widely used in culinary traditions and herbal medicine, cloves are rich in antioxidants and essential oils with potential health benefits. Incorporating clove tea into a diabetes management plan offers a delicious and natural way to support blood sugar control and overall well-being.

Health Benefits of Clove Tea:

Cloves are rich in antioxidants, including eugenol, which has been studied for its potential anti-inflammatory and blood sugar-regulating properties.
The essential oils present in cloves may help improve digestion and alleviate gastrointestinal discomfort.

Impact on Blood Sugar Regulation:
Studies suggest that eugenol, the main
component of clove oil, may help improve
insulin sensitivity and regulate blood sugar
levels.
By incorporating clove tea into a diabetes
management plan, individuals may benefit from
the potential blood sugar-lowering effects of
this aromatic spice.

How to Prepare Clove Tea:

Ingredients:
1 cup of water
3-4 whole cloves
Sweetener of choice (optional).

Instructions:
Heat the water in a small saucepan until it
boils.
Add the whole cloves to the boiling water.
Reduce the heat and simmer the tea for 5-10
minutes to allow the flavors to infuse.

Remove the saucepan from the heat and let the clove tea steep for a few minutes.
Strain the clove tea into cups, add sweetener if desired, and enjoy.

Variations of Clove Tea:
Clove Cinnamon Tea: Add a cinnamon stick to the clove tea for a warm and spicy flavor combination.
Clove Lemon Tea: Squeeze a fresh lemon wedge into the clove tea for a citrusy twist and add vitamin C.

Incorporating Clove Tea into a Diabetes Management Plan:
Enjoying clove tea as part of a balanced diet and lifestyle can provide a flavorful and healthful way to support blood sugar control and overall well-being.
Be mindful of added sweeteners, especially for individuals managing carbohydrate intake.

Precautions and Considerations:
Clove tea is generally safe for consumption, but individuals with certain medical conditions or allergies should consult with a healthcare provider before incorporating it into their diet. Monitor blood sugar levels regularly and adjust clove tea consumption as needed based on individual response.

Clove tea offers a fragrant and aromatic beverage option for individuals managing diabetes. With its rich antioxidants and potential blood sugar-regulating properties, clove tea provides a flavorful and healthful addition to a diabetes management plan. By incorporating clove tea into their daily routines, individuals can enjoy its potential benefits for blood sugar control and overall well-being, all while savoring it's comforting and aromatic flavors

Black Pepper Tea

Black pepper tea is a warm and invigorating beverage made by steeping black peppercorns in hot water. Widely used in culinary traditions and Ayurvedic medicine, black pepper is known for its distinct flavor and potential health benefits. Incorporating black pepper tea into a diabetes management plan offers a flavorful and natural way to support blood sugar control and overall well-being.

Health Benefits of Black Pepper Tea:
Black pepper contains piperine, a compound with antioxidant and anti-inflammatory properties that may contribute to its potential health benefits.
Piperine has been studied for its potential to improve digestion, enhance nutrient absorption, and regulate blood sugar levels.

Impact on Blood Sugar Regulation:
Studies suggest that piperine, the active compound in black pepper, may help improve insulin sensitivity and regulate blood sugar levels.
By incorporating black pepper tea into a diabetes management plan, individuals may benefit from the potential blood sugar-lowering effects of this aromatic spice.

How to Prepare Black Pepper Tea:

Ingredients:
1 cup of water
1 teaspoon of whole black peppercorns
Sweetener of choice (optional)

Instructions:
In a small saucepan, bring the water to a boil.
Add the whole black peppercorns to the boiling water.

Reduce the heat and simmer the tea for 5-10 minutes to allow the flavors to infuse.
Remove the saucepan from the heat and let the black pepper tea steep for a few minutes.
Strain the tea into cups, add sweetener if desired, and enjoy.

Variations of Black Pepper Tea:
Black Pepper Lemon Tea: Squeeze a fresh lemon wedge into the black pepper tea for a citrusy twist and add vitamin C.
Black Pepper Ginger Tea: Add a few slices of fresh ginger to the black pepper tea for a spicy and warming flavor combination.

Incorporating Black Pepper Tea into a Diabetes Management Plan:
Enjoying black pepper tea as part of a balanced diet and lifestyle can provide a flavorful and healthful way to support blood sugar control and overall well-being.
Be mindful of added sweeteners, especially for individuals managing carbohydrate intake.

Precautions and Considerations:
Black pepper tea is generally safe for consumption, but individuals with certain medical conditions or allergies should consult with a healthcare provider before incorporating it into their diet.
Monitor blood sugar levels regularly and adjust black pepper tea consumption as needed based on individual response.

Black pepper tea offers a warm and aromatic beverage option for individuals managing diabetes. With its potential blood sugar-regulating properties and distinct flavor, black pepper tea provides a flavorful and healthful addition to a diabetes management plan. By incorporating black pepper tea into their daily routines, individuals can enjoy its potential benefits for blood sugar control and overall well-being, all while savoring its invigorating and aromatic flavors.

Masala Tea

Masala tea, also known as spiced tea or chai masala, is a popular beverage originating from the Indian subcontinent. This aromatic tea is made by infusing black tea with a blend of spices, creating a flavorful and invigorating drink. Incorporating masala tea into a diabetes management plan offers a delicious and natural way to support blood sugar control and overall well-being, while also enjoying the rich flavors of traditional spices.

Health Benefits of Masala Tea:
Masala tea contains a variety of spices, each offering potential health benefits. Common spices used in masala tea include cinnamon, cardamom, cloves, ginger, and black pepper. These spices are rich in antioxidants and bioactive compounds that may help improve digestion, reduce inflammation, and regulate blood sugar levels.

Impact on Blood Sugar Regulation:
The spices found in masala tea, such as
cinnamon and ginger, have been studied for
their potential to improve insulin sensitivity and
regulate blood sugar levels.
By incorporating masala tea into a diabetes
management plan, individuals may benefit from
the potential blood sugar-lowering effects of
these spices.

How to Prepare Masala Tea:

Ingredients:
1 cup of water
1 black tea bag or 1 tablespoon of loose black
tea leaves
Spices: cinnamon stick, cardamom pods,
cloves, ginger slices, black peppercorns
Milk (dairy or plant-based)
Sweetener of choice (optional).

Instructions:

In a small saucepan, bring the water to a boil.
Add the black tea bag or tea leaves to the
boiling water.
Add the spices to the saucepan, adjusting the
quantities to suit your taste preferences.
Simmer the tea and spices for 3-5 minutes to
allow the flavors to infuse.
Add milk to the saucepan and continue to
simmer for an additional 2-3 minutes.
Remove the saucepan from the heat and let
the masala tea steep for a few minutes.
Strain the tea into cups, add sweetener if
desired, and enjoy.

Variations of Masala Tea:

Decaffeinated Masala Tea: Use decaffeinated
black tea to reduce caffeine intake, especially
for those sensitive to caffeine.
Masala Green Tea: Substitute black tea with
green tea for a lighter and more delicate flavor
profile.

Incorporating Masala Tea into a Diabetes Management Plan:
Enjoying masala tea as part of a balanced diet and lifestyle can provide a flavorful and healthful way to support blood sugar control and overall well-being.
Be mindful of added sweeteners and high-fat milk content, especially for individuals managing carbohydrate and fat intake.

Precautions and Considerations:
Individuals with gastrointestinal issues or sensitivities to spices should consume masala tea in moderation.
Monitor blood sugar levels regularly and adjust masala tea consumption as needed based on individual response.

Masala tea offers a fragrant and aromatic beverage option for individuals managing diabetes. With its blend of spices and black tea, masala tea provides a flavorful and healthful addition to a diabetes management plan. By incorporating masala tea into their daily routines, individuals can enjoy its potential benefits for blood sugar control and overall well-being, all while savoring its aromatic and invigorating flavors.

CHAPTER SIX

Antioxidant-rich Tea Elixirs for Diabetes Support

Antioxidant-rich tea elixirs offer a flavorful and healthful way to support blood sugar management and overall well-being for individuals with diabetes. By combining various teas with antioxidant-rich ingredients, these elixirs provide a delicious alternative to traditional beverages while harnessing the potential health benefits of antioxidants. Incorporating antioxidant-rich tea elixirs into a diabetes management plan can add variety to the diet and contribute to improved blood sugar control.

Health Benefits of Antioxidant-Rich Tea Elixirs:

Antioxidants found in tea, herbs, and spices have been studied for their potential to reduce oxidative stress, inflammation, and improve insulin sensitivity.

By incorporating antioxidant-rich ingredients into tea elixirs, individuals may benefit from enhanced immune function, improved cardiovascular health, and better blood sugar regulation.

Popular Antioxidant-Rich Ingredients for Tea Elixirs:

Green Tea: Rich in catechins such as epigallocatechin gallate (EGCG), green tea offers potent antioxidant properties that may support blood sugar control and reduce the risk of complications associated with diabetes.

Herbs and Spices: Ingredients like cinnamon, ginger, turmeric, and cloves are rich in antioxidants and bioactive compounds that have been shown to have beneficial effects on blood sugar levels and overall health.
Citrus Fruits: Adding citrus fruits like lemon or orange to tea elixirs provides a boost of vitamin C and flavonoids, which have antioxidant and anti-inflammatory properties.

How to Prepare Antioxidant-Rich Tea Elixirs:

Ingredients:
Choice of tea base (green tea, black tea, herbal tea)
Antioxidant-rich ingredients (cinnamon sticks, ginger slices, turmeric powder, cloves, citrus fruits)
Hot water
Sweetener of choice (optional).

Instructions:

Brew the tea base according to package instructions or personal preference.

Add antioxidant-rich ingredients to the brewed tea, such as cinnamon sticks, ginger slices, turmeric powder, cloves, or citrus fruits.

Allow the tea and ingredients to steep for a few minutes to infuse flavors and release antioxidants.

Strain the tea elixir into cups, add sweetener if desired, and enjoy.

Variations of Antioxidant-Rich Tea Elixirs:

Citrus Green Tea Elixir: Brew green tea and add fresh lemon slices for a refreshing and antioxidant-rich beverage.

Spiced Herbal Tea Elixir: Use herbal tea as a base and add cinnamon, ginger, and cloves for a warming and flavorful elixir.

Turmeric Ginger Tea Elixir: Combine green tea with turmeric powder and ginger slices for a soothing and antioxidant-packed elixir.

Incorporating Antioxidant-Rich Tea Elixirs into a Diabetes Management Plan:
Enjoying antioxidant-rich tea elixirs as part of a balanced diet and lifestyle can provide a flavorful and healthful way to support blood sugar control and overall well-being.
Aim to include antioxidant-rich tea elixirs as a regular beverage option, alongside other diabetes-friendly choices.

Precautions and Considerations:
Individuals with certain medical conditions or allergies should consult with a healthcare provider before incorporating antioxidant-rich tea elixirs into their diet.
Monitor blood sugar levels regularly and adjust consumption as needed based on individual response.

Antioxidant-rich tea elixirs offer a delicious and healthful option for individuals managing diabetes. By combining tea bases with antioxidant-rich ingredients like herbs, spices, and citrus fruits, these elixirs provide a flavorful and beneficial addition to a diabetes management plan. By incorporating antioxidant-rich tea elixirs into their daily routines, individuals can enjoy their potential benefits for blood sugar control and overall well-being, all while savoring their aromatic and invigorating flavors.

Rooibos Tea

Rooibos tea, also known as red bush tea, is a popular herbal infusion brewed from the leaves of the Aspalathus linearis plant, native to South Africa. Renowned for its distinct flavor, vibrant red color, and potential health benefits, rooibos tea has gained popularity worldwide. Incorporating rooibos tea into a diabetes management plan offers a flavorful and healthful way to support blood sugar control and overall well-being.

Health Benefits of Rooibos Tea:

Antioxidant Richness: Rooibos tea is abundant in antioxidants, such as and nothofagin, which may help reduce oxidative stress and inflammation, factors associated with diabetes and its complications.

Caffeine-Free: Unlike traditional teas like green or black tea, rooibos tea is naturally caffeine-free, making it a suitable option for individuals sensitive to caffeine or those looking to reduce their caffeine intake.

Hydration: Staying hydrated is essential for overall health, including diabetes management. Rooibos tea provides a hydrating alternative to sugary or caffeinated beverages.

Impact on Blood Sugar Regulation:
While specific research on rooibos tea's effects on blood sugar regulation is limited, its antioxidant properties may indirectly support diabetes management. By reducing oxidative stress and inflammation, rooibos tea may contribute to improved insulin sensitivity and overall blood sugar control.

Flavor Profile and Preparation:

Mild and Nutty Flavor: Rooibos tea boasts a naturally mild and slightly sweet flavor profile with nutty undertones, making it a versatile beverage suitable for various palates.

Preparation: Brewing rooibos tea is simple. Steep rooibos tea leaves or tea bags in hot water for 5-7 minutes, allowing the flavors to infuse fully. Strain and serve plain or with a splash of milk and a touch of sweetener, according to preference.

Variations of Rooibos Tea:

Rooibos Chai: Infuse rooibos tea with traditional chai spices like cinnamon, cardamom, cloves, and ginger for a warming and aromatic beverage.

Rooibos Citrus: Enhance brewed rooibos tea with a squeeze of fresh lemon or orange for a refreshing and citrusy twist.

Rooibos Mint: Add a burst of freshness to brewed rooibos tea by garnishing it with fresh mint leaves, perfect for a cool and invigorating flavor.

Incorporating Rooibos Tea into a Diabetes Management Plan:

Regular Consumption: Enjoying rooibos tea regularly as part of a balanced diet and lifestyle can provide a flavorful and healthful way to support blood sugar control and overall well-being.

Hydration Alternative: Rooibos tea can serve as a hydrating alternative to sugary beverages, helping individuals stay hydrated without the added sugars and calories.

Precautions and Considerations:

Consultation: Individuals with specific medical conditions or allergies should consult with a healthcare provider before incorporating rooibos tea into their diet.

Monitoring: Regular monitoring of blood sugar levels is crucial, allowing individuals to adjust rooibos tea consumption as needed based on individual responses.

Rooibos tea presents a flavorful and healthful beverage option for individuals managing diabetes. With its antioxidant-rich properties, caffeine-free nature, and versatile flavor profile, rooibos tea can complement a diabetes management plan effectively. By incorporating rooibos tea into their daily routines, individuals can enjoy its potential benefits for blood sugar control and overall well-being, all while savoring its unique flavor and soothing qualities.

Hibiscus Tea

Hibiscus tea is a vibrant and tangy herbal infusion made from the dried calyces of the Hibiscus flower. With its bold red color and refreshing taste, hibiscus tea is not only delicious but also offers potential health benefits, making it a valuable addition to a diabetes management plan.

Health Benefits of Hibiscus Tea:

Antioxidant Richness: Hibiscus tea is packed with antioxidants, including flavonoids and polyphenols, which help combat oxidative stress and inflammation, contributing to overall health and well-being.

Blood Pressure Management: Studies suggest that hibiscus tea may help lower blood pressure levels, which is beneficial for individuals with diabetes who are at higher risk of hypertension.

Blood Sugar Control: Research indicates that hibiscus tea consumption may help lower blood sugar levels by improving insulin sensitivity and reducing blood sugar absorption.

Impact on Blood Sugar Regulation:
Hibiscus tea's potential to lower blood sugar levels makes it particularly beneficial for individuals with diabetes. The antioxidants and bioactive compounds found in hibiscus tea may help improve insulin sensitivity and regulate blood sugar levels, contributing to better glycemic control.

Flavor Profile and Preparation:

Tangy and Refreshing: Hibiscus tea has a tangy and slightly tart flavor profile with subtle floral notes, making it a refreshing beverage option.

Preparation: To prepare hibiscus tea, steep dried hibiscus flowers or tea bags in hot water for 5-10 minutes, allowing the flavors to infuse fully. Strain and serve plain or with a touch of honey for sweetness, if desired.

Variations of Hibiscus Tea:

Hibiscus Ginger Tea: Add freshly sliced ginger to brewed hibiscus tea for a spicy and invigorating flavor combination, which may also aid digestion.

Hibiscus Mint Tea: Garnish brewed hibiscus tea with fresh mint leaves for a cool and refreshing twist, perfect for hot summer days.

Including Hibiscus Tea in a Plan for Managing Diabetes:

Regular Consumption: Enjoying hibiscus tea as part of a balanced diet and lifestyle can provide a flavorful and healthful way to support blood sugar control and overall well-being.

Hydration Alternative: Hibiscus tea can serve as a hydrating alternative to sugary beverages, helping individuals stay hydrated without the added sugars and calories.

Precautions and Considerations:

Consultation: Individuals taking medications for blood pressure or diabetes should consult with a healthcare provider before incorporating hibiscus tea into their diet, as it may interact with certain medications.

Monitoring: Regular monitoring of blood sugar levels is essential, allowing individuals to adjust hibiscus tea consumption as needed based on individual responses.

Hibiscus tea offers a tangy and refreshing beverage option for individuals managing diabetes. With its antioxidant-rich properties and potential benefits for blood sugar control and blood pressure management, hibiscus tea can play a valuable role in a diabetes management plan. By incorporating hibiscus tea into their daily routines, individuals can enjoy its potential health benefits while savoring its delightful flavor profile.

Elderberry Tea

Elderberry tea is a soothing and flavorful herbal infusion made from the dried elderberry fruit of the Sambucus nigra plant. With its rich purple color and sweet-tart flavor, elderberry tea offers not only a delightful drinking experience but also potential health benefits that can support diabetes management.

Health Benefits of Elderberry Tea:

Antioxidant Powerhouse: Elderberries are loaded with antioxidants, particularly flavonoids like quercetin and anthocyanins, which help combat oxidative stress and inflammation in the body.

Immune Support: Elderberry tea is renowned for its immune-boosting properties, which can help individuals with diabetes maintain overall health and well-being.

Heart Health: Some studies suggest that elderberries may help improve cardiovascular health by lowering cholesterol levels and supporting healthy blood vessel function.

Impact on Blood Sugar Regulation:
While specific research on elderberry tea's effects on blood sugar regulation is limited, its antioxidant-rich profile and potential anti-inflammatory properties may indirectly support diabetes management. By reducing oxidative stress and inflammation, elderberry tea may contribute to improved insulin sensitivity and overall blood sugar control.

Flavor Profile and Preparation:

Sweet-Tart Flavor: Elderberry tea boasts a sweet-tart flavor profile with floral undertones, making it a delicious and refreshing beverage option.

Preparation: To prepare elderberry tea, steep dried elderberries for elderberry tea bags in hot water for 10-15 minutes, allowing the flavors to infuse fully. Strain and serve plain or with a touch of honey for sweetness, if desired.

Variations of Elderberry Tea:

Elderberry Ginger Tea: Add freshly sliced ginger to brewed elderberry tea for a spicy and invigorating flavor combination, which may also aid digestion and provide additional immune support.

Elderberry Lemon Tea: Enhance brewed elderberry tea with a squeeze of fresh lemon for a bright and citrusy twist, perfect for boosting vitamin C intake and adding a refreshing flavor.

**Incorporating Elderberry Tea into a
Diabetes Management Plan:**

Regular Consumption: Enjoying elderberry
tea as part of a balanced diet and lifestyle can
provide a flavorful and healthful way to support
overall health and potentially aid in diabetes
management.

Hydration Alternative: Elderberry tea can
serve as a hydrating alternative to sugary
beverages, helping individuals stay hydrated
without the added sugars and calories.

Precautions and Considerations:

Consultation: Individuals with certain medical
conditions or allergies should consult with a
healthcare provider before incorporating
elderberry tea into their diet, especially if they
are taking medications or supplements.

Monitoring: Regular monitoring of blood sugar levels is essential, allowing individuals to adjust elderberry tea consumption as needed based on individual responses.

Elderberry tea offers a flavorful and healthful beverage option for individuals managing diabetes. With its antioxidant-rich properties and potential benefits for immune support and overall health, elderberry tea can be a valuable addition to a diabetes management plan. By incorporating elderberry tea into their daily routines, individuals can enjoy its delightful flavor and potential health benefits while supporting their overall well-being.

Cranberry Tea

Cranberry tea is a tart and refreshing herbal infusion made from the dried cranberries of the Vaccinium plant. Renowned for its vibrant red color and tangy flavor, cranberry tea not only offers a delightful drinking experience but also potential health benefits that can support diabetes management.

Health Benefits of Cranberry Tea:

Urinary Tract Health: Cranberries contain compounds called proanthocyanidins, which may help prevent urinary tract infections (UTIs) by preventing bacteria from adhering to the walls of the urinary tract.

Antioxidant Properties: Cranberries are rich in antioxidants, particularly flavonoids and polyphenols, which help combat oxidative stress and inflammation in the body.

Heart Health: Some studies suggest that cranberries may help improve cardiovascular health by reducing LDL cholesterol levels and supporting healthy blood vessel function.

Impact on Blood Sugar Regulation:
While specific research on cranberry tea's effects on blood sugar regulation is limited, its antioxidant-rich profile and potential anti-inflammatory properties may indirectly support diabetes management. By reducing oxidative stress and inflammation, cranberry tea may contribute to improved insulin sensitivity and overall blood sugar control.

Flavor Profile and Preparation:

Tart and Refreshing: Cranberry tea boasts a tart and slightly sour flavor profile, making it a refreshing and invigorating beverage option.

Preparation: To prepare cranberry tea, steep dried cranberries or cranberry tea bags in hot water for 10-15 minutes, allowing the flavors to infuse fully. Strain and serve plain or with a touch of honey for sweetness, if desired.

Variations of Cranberry Tea:

Cranberry Orange Tea: Enhance brewed cranberry tea with a twist of fresh orange zest for a citrusy and aromatic flavor combination, perfect for brightening up your day.

Cranberry Cinnamon Tea: Add a cinnamon stick to brewed cranberry tea for a warm and comforting flavor profile, reminiscent of the holiday season.

**Incorporating Cranberry Tea into a Diabetes
Management Plan:**

Regular Consumption: Enjoying cranberry
tea as part of a balanced diet and lifestyle can
provide a flavorful and healthful way to support
urinary tract health and potentially aid in
diabetes management.

Hydration Alternative: Cranberry tea can
serve as a hydrating alternative to sugary
beverages, helping individuals stay hydrated
without the added sugars and calories.

Precautions and Considerations:

Consultation: Individuals with certain medical
conditions or allergies should consult with a
healthcare provider before incorporating
cranberry tea into their diet, especially if they
are taking medications or supplements.

Monitoring: Regular monitoring of blood sugar levels is essential, allowing individuals to adjust cranberry tea consumption as needed based on individual responses.

Cranberry tea offers a tart and refreshing beverage option for individuals managing diabetes. With its potential benefits for urinary tract health and overall well-being, cranberry tea can be a valuable addition to a diabetes management plan. By incorporating cranberry tea into their daily routines, individuals can enjoy its delightful flavor and potential health benefits while supporting their overall health and well-being.

Blueberry Tea

Blueberry tea is a delightful and flavorful herbal infusion made from the dried blueberries of the Vaccinium plant. With its deep blue color and sweet-tart flavor, blueberry tea not only offers a delicious drinking experience but also potential health benefits that can support diabetes management.

Health Benefits of Blueberry Tea:

Antioxidant Powerhouse: Blueberries are rich in antioxidants, particularly anthocyanins, which help combat oxidative stress and inflammation in the body.

Heart Health: Studies suggest that blueberries may help improve cardiovascular health by reducing LDL cholesterol levels and supporting healthy blood vessel function.

Cognitive Function: Some research indicates that the antioxidants in blueberries may help protect brain cells from damage and improve cognitive function, which is important for overall well-being.

Impact on Blood Sugar Regulation:
While specific research on blueberry tea's effects on blood sugar regulation is limited, its antioxidant-rich profile and potential anti-inflammatory properties may indirectly support diabetes management. By reducing oxidative stress and inflammation, blueberry tea may contribute to improved insulin sensitivity and overall blood sugar control.

Flavor Profile and Preparation:

Sweet and Tart: Blueberry tea boasts a sweet and slightly tart flavor profile, making it a refreshing and enjoyable beverage option.

Preparation: To prepare blueberry tea, steep dried blueberries or blueberry tea bags in hot water for 10-15 minutes, allowing the flavors to infuse fully. Strain and serve plain or with a touch of honey for sweetness, if desired.

Variations of Blueberry Tea:

Blueberry Lemon Tea: Enhance brewed blueberry tea with a squeeze of fresh lemon for a bright and citrusy flavor combination, perfect for refreshing the palate.

Blueberry Mint Tea: Add fresh mint leaves to brewed blueberry tea for a cool and invigorating twist, providing a burst of freshness with every sip.

Incorporating Blueberry Tea into a Diabetes Management Plan:

Regular Consumption: Enjoying blueberry tea as part of a balanced diet and lifestyle can provide a flavorful and healthful way to support overall well-being and potentially aid in diabetes management.

Hydration Alternative: Blueberry tea can serve as a hydrating alternative to sugary beverages, helping individuals stay hydrated without the added sugars and calories.

Precautions and Considerations:

Consultation: Individuals with certain medical conditions or allergies should consult with a healthcare provider before incorporating blueberry tea into their diet, especially if they are taking medications or supplements.

Monitoring: Regular monitoring of blood sugar levels is essential, allowing individuals to adjust blueberry tea consumption as needed based on individual responses.

Blueberry tea offers a delicious and healthful beverage option for individuals managing diabetes. With its antioxidant-rich properties and potential benefits for overall well-being, blueberry tea can be a valuable addition to a diabetes management plan. By incorporating blueberry tea into their daily routines, individuals can enjoy its delightful flavor and potential health benefits while supporting their overall health and well-being.

CHAPTER SEVEN

Herbal Remedies and Tea Combinations for Insulin Sensitivity

Herbal remedies and tea combinations can play a significant role in improving insulin sensitivity, a crucial aspect of diabetes management. By incorporating specific herbs and teas known for their insulin-sensitizing properties into one's daily routine, individuals with diabetes can support better blood sugar control and overall health.

Herbal Remedies for Insulin Sensitivity:

Cinnamon: Cinnamon is well-known for its ability to improve insulin sensitivity and lower blood sugar levels. Adding cinnamon to tea blends or consuming cinnamon tea regularly can be beneficial for individuals with diabetes.

Fenugreek: Fenugreek seeds contain soluble fiber and compounds that may help improve insulin sensitivity and reduce blood sugar levels. Brewing fenugreek tea or adding fenugreek seeds to herbal tea blends can support diabetes management.

Ginger: Ginger has anti-inflammatory properties and may help enhance insulin sensitivity. Adding fresh ginger slices to tea or brewing ginger tea can aid in blood sugar regulation.

Turmeric: Curcumin, the active compound in turmeric, has been studied for its potential to improve insulin sensitivity and reduce inflammation. Brewing turmeric tea or adding turmeric powder to herbal tea blends can provide these benefits.

Tea Combinations for Insulin Sensitivity:

Cinnamon Ginger Tea: Combine cinnamon and ginger in a tea blend for a flavorful and insulin-sensitizing beverage that supports blood sugar control and digestion.

Fenugreek Turmeric Tea: Blend fenugreek seeds and turmeric powder to create a tea rich in soluble fiber and anti-inflammatory compounds, promoting better insulin sensitivity and overall health.

Cinnamon Fenugreek Tea: Brew a combination of cinnamon and fenugreek seeds for a potent herbal tea that aids in improving insulin sensitivity and lowering blood sugar levels.

Ginger Turmeric Tea: Combine ginger and turmeric in a tea blend for a warming and anti-inflammatory beverage that supports better insulin sensitivity and overall well-being.

Incorporating Herbal Remedies and Tea Combinations into a Diabetes Management Plan:

Regular Consumption: Enjoying herbal remedies and tea combinations as part of a balanced diet and lifestyle can provide a flavorful and healthful way to support insulin sensitivity and overall blood sugar control.

Variety and Experimentation: Explore different herbal remedies and tea combinations to find what works best for individual preferences and needs. Incorporate a variety of herbs and teas into daily routines for maximum benefits.

Precautions and Considerations:

Consultation: Individuals with diabetes should consult with a healthcare provider before incorporating herbal remedies and tea combinations into their diet, especially if they are taking medications or supplements.

Monitoring: Regular monitoring of blood sugar levels is essential to assess the effects of herbal remedies and tea combinations on insulin sensitivity and overall diabetes management.

Herbal remedies and tea combinations offer a natural and effective way to improve insulin sensitivity and support diabetes management. By incorporating specific herbs and teas known for their insulin-sensitizing properties into one's daily routine, individuals with diabetes can enhance blood sugar control and promote overall well-being. With a variety of flavorful options to choose from, herbal remedies and tea combinations can be enjoyed as part of a holistic approach to diabetes care.

Holy Basil Tea

Holy Basil, also known as Tulsi, is a sacred herb in Ayurvedic medicine and is revered for its numerous health benefits, including its potential to support diabetes management. Brewing Holy Basil tea offers a flavorful and healthful beverage option for individuals seeking to improve blood sugar control and overall well-being.

Health Benefits of Holy Basil Tea:

Blood Sugar Regulation: Holy Basil contains compounds like eugenol and triterpenoids, which may help lower blood sugar levels by increasing insulin sensitivity and stimulating insulin secretion from the pancreas.

Antioxidant Properties: Holy Basil is rich in antioxidants, such as flavonoids and polyphenols, which help combat oxidative stress and inflammation in the body, contributing to better overall health.

Stress Reduction: Holy Basil is considered an adaptogen, meaning it helps the body adapt to stress. By reducing stress levels, Holy Basil may indirectly support diabetes management, as stress hormones can affect blood sugar levels.

Impact on Blood Sugar Regulation:
Research suggests that Holy Basil may help lower blood sugar levels and improve insulin sensitivity, making it a valuable herb for individuals with diabetes. By incorporating Holy Basil tea into a diabetes management plan, individuals can potentially experience better blood sugar control and overall health.

Flavor Profile and Preparation:

Refreshing and Herbal: Holy Basil tea has a refreshing and herbal flavor profile with hints of mint and spice, making it a soothing and enjoyable beverage option.

Preparation: To prepare Holy Basil tea, steep fresh or dried Holy Basil leaves in hot water for 5-10 minutes, allowing the flavors to infuse fully. Strain and serve plain or with a touch of honey for sweetness, if desired.

Variations of Holy Basil Tea:

Holy Basil Lemon Tea: Enhance brewed Holy Basil tea with a squeeze of fresh lemon for a citrusy and aromatic flavor combination, perfect for refreshing the palate.

Holy Basil Ginger Tea: Add freshly sliced ginger to brewed Holy Basil tea for a spicy and invigorating twist, which may also aid digestion and provide additional health benefits.

Incorporating Holy Basil Tea into a Diabetes Management Plan:

Regular Consumption: Enjoying Holy Basil tea as part of a balanced diet and lifestyle can provide a flavorful and healthful way to support blood sugar control and overall well-being.

Hydration Alternative: Holy Basil tea can serve as a hydrating alternative to sugary beverages, helping individuals stay hydrated without the added sugars and calories.

Precautions and Considerations:

Consultation: Individuals with certain medical conditions or allergies should consult with a healthcare provider before incorporating Holy Basil tea into their diet, especially if they are taking medications or supplements.

Monitoring: Regular monitoring of blood sugar levels is essential, allowing individuals to assess the effects of Holy Basil tea on blood sugar regulation and adjust consumption as needed.

Holy Basil tea offers a flavorful and healthful beverage option for individuals managing diabetes. With its potential benefits for blood sugar regulation, antioxidant properties, and stress reduction, Holy Basil tea can be a valuable addition to a diabetes management plan. By incorporating Holy Basil tea into their daily routines, individuals can enjoy its delightful flavor and potential health benefits while supporting their overall health and well-being.

Nettle Leaf Tea

Nettle leaf tea, brewed from the leaves of the stinging nettle plant, offers a unique herbal infusion with potential health benefits, including support for diabetes management. With its earthy flavor and nutrient-rich profile, nettle leaf tea provides a flavorful and healthful beverage option for individuals seeking to improve blood sugar control and overall well-being.

Health Benefits of Nettle Leaf Tea:

Blood Sugar Regulation: Nettle leaf contains compounds that may help regulate blood sugar levels by improving insulin sensitivity and reducing inflammation in the body.

Nutrient Density: Nettle leaf is rich in vitamins, minerals, and antioxidants, including vitamins A, C, and K, iron, and calcium, which support overall health and well-being.

Anti-inflammatory Properties: Nettle leaf possesses anti-inflammatory properties, which may help reduce inflammation in the body and alleviate symptoms associated with diabetes and other chronic conditions.

Impact on Blood Sugar Regulation:
Research suggests that the compounds found in nettle leaf may help improve insulin sensitivity and regulate blood sugar levels, making nettle leaf tea a valuable addition to a diabetes management plan. By incorporating nettle leaf tea into their daily routine, individuals with diabetes may experience better blood sugar control and overall health.

Flavor Profile and Preparation:

Earthy and Mild: Nettle leaf tea has an earthy and mildly grassy flavor profile, with subtle notes of sweetness. It is soothing and refreshing, making it a pleasant beverage choice.

Preparation: To prepare nettle leaf tea, steep dried nettle leaves in hot water for 5-10 minutes, allowing the flavors to infuse fully. Strain and serve plain or with a touch of honey for sweetness, if desired.

Variations of Nettle Leaf Tea:

Nettle Peppermint Tea: Blend dried nettle leaves with peppermint leaves for a refreshing and invigorating tea blend that supports digestion and provides additional health benefits.

Nettle Lemon Ginger Tea: Add freshly sliced ginger and a squeeze of fresh lemon to brewed nettle leaf tea for a zesty and aromatic beverage that aids in digestion and enhances flavor.

Incorporating Nettle Leaf Tea into a Diabetes Management Plan:

Regular Consumption: Enjoying nettle leaf tea as part of a balanced diet and lifestyle can provide a flavorful and healthful way to support blood sugar control and overall well-being.

Hydration Alternative: Nettle leaf tea can serve as a hydrating alternative to sugary beverages, helping individuals stay hydrated without the added sugars and calories.

Precautions and Considerations:

Consultation: Individuals with certain medical conditions or allergies should consult with a healthcare provider before incorporating nettle leaf tea into their diet, especially if they are taking medications or supplements.

Monitoring: Regular monitoring of blood sugar levels is essential, allowing individuals to assess the effects of nettle leaf tea on blood sugar regulation and adjust consumption as needed.

Nettle leaf tea offers a flavorful and healthful beverage option for individuals managing diabetes. With its potential benefits for blood sugar regulation, nutrient density, and anti-inflammatory properties, nettle leaf tea can be a valuable addition to a diabetes management plan. By incorporating nettle leaf tea into their daily routines, individuals can enjoy its delightful flavor and potential health benefits while supporting their overall health and well-being.

Dandelion Root Tea

Dandelion root tea, brewed from the dried roots of the common dandelion plant, offers a flavorful and healthful herbal infusion with potential benefits for individuals managing diabetes. With its earthy flavor and nutritional richness, dandelion root tea provides a satisfying beverage option that may support blood sugar control and overall well-being.

Health Benefits of Dandelion Root Tea:

Blood Sugar Regulation: Dandelion root contains compounds that may help regulate blood sugar levels by improving insulin sensitivity and reducing inflammation in the body.

Liver Support: Dandelion root is believed to support liver health by promoting detoxification and aiding in the elimination of waste products from the body, which can benefit individuals with diabetes who may experience liver-related complications.

Digestive Health: Dandelion root has traditionally been used to support digestive health by stimulating appetite, promoting healthy digestion, and relieving symptoms of bloating and indigestion.

Impact on Blood Sugar Regulation:
While specific research on dandelion root tea's effects on blood sugar regulation is limited, its potential to improve insulin sensitivity and support liver health may indirectly benefit individuals managing diabetes. By incorporating dandelion root tea into their daily routine, individuals may experience better blood sugar control and overall health.

Flavor Profile and Preparation:

Earthy and Nutty: Dandelion root tea has an earthy and slightly nutty flavor profile, with hints of bitterness. It is grounding and comforting, making it a satisfying beverage choice.

Preparation: To prepare dandelion root tea, steep dried dandelion roots in hot water for 5-10 minutes, allowing the flavors to infuse fully. Strain and serve plain or with a touch of honey for sweetness, if desired.

Variations of Dandelion Root Tea:

Dandelion Root Ginger Tea: Add freshly sliced ginger to brewed dandelion root tea for a spicy and invigorating flavor combination that aids in digestion and enhances the overall taste.

Dandelion Root Cinnamon Tea: Blend brewed dandelion root tea with a dash of cinnamon for a warming and aromatic beverage that adds depth to the flavor profile and may provide additional health benefits.

Incorporating Dandelion Root Tea into a Diabetes Management Plan:

Regular Consumption: Enjoying dandelion root tea as part of a balanced diet and lifestyle can provide a flavorful and healthful way to support blood sugar control and overall well-being.

Hydration Alternative: Dandelion root tea can serve as a hydrating alternative to sugary beverages, helping individuals stay hydrated without the added sugars and calories.

Precautions and Considerations:

Consultation: Individuals with certain medical conditions or allergies should consult with a healthcare provider before incorporating dandelion root tea into their diet, especially if they are taking medications or supplements.

Monitoring: Regular monitoring of blood sugar levels is essential, allowing individuals to assess the effects of dandelion root tea on blood sugar regulation and adjust consumption as needed.

Dandelion root tea offers a flavorful and healthful beverage option for individuals managing diabetes. With its potential benefits for blood sugar regulation, liver support, and digestive health, dandelion root tea can be a valuable addition to a diabetes management plan.

Gymnema Sylvestre Tea

Gymnema Sylvestre, also known as the "sugar destroyer," is a woody climbing shrub native to India and Africa. Gymnema Sylvestre tea, brewed from the leaves of this plant, has been used for centuries in traditional Ayurvedic medicine to support diabetes management. With its unique ability to reduce sugar cravings and potentially improve blood sugar control, Gymnema Sylvestre tea offers a flavorful and healthful beverage option for individuals with diabetes.

Health Benefits of Gymnema Sylvestre Tea:

Blood Sugar Regulation: Gymnema Sylvestre contains compounds called acids, which may help lower blood sugar levels by blocking sugar absorption in the intestines and improving insulin sensitivity.

Reduced Sugar Cravings: Gymnema Sylvestre has a unique ability to temporarily suppress the taste of sweetness, reducing sugar cravings and potentially promoting healthier eating habits for individuals with diabetes.

Weight Management: By reducing sugar cravings and potentially improving blood sugar control, Gymnema Sylvestre tea may support weight management efforts, as excess weight can worsen diabetes symptoms.

Impact on Blood Sugar Regulation: Research suggests that Gymnema Sylvestre tea may help improve blood sugar control by reducing sugar absorption in the intestines and increasing insulin sensitivity. By incorporating Gymnema Sylvestre tea into their daily routine, individuals with diabetes may experience better blood sugar regulation and overall health.

Flavor Profile and Preparation:

Earthy and Bitter: Gymnema Sylvestre tea has an earthy and slightly bitter flavor profile, with subtle herbal undertones. It is grounding and soothing, making it a satisfying beverage choice.

Preparation: To prepare Gymnema Sylvestre tea, steep dried Gymnema Sylvestre leaves in hot water for 5-10 minutes, allowing the flavors to infuse fully. Strain and serve plain or with a touch of honey for sweetness, if desired.

Incorporating Gymnema Sylvestre Tea into a Diabetes Management Plan:

Regular Consumption: Enjoying Gymnema Sylvestre tea as part of a balanced diet and lifestyle can provide a flavorful and healthful way to support blood sugar control and reduce sugar cravings.

Hydration Alternative: Gymnema Sylvestre tea can serve as a hydrating alternative to sugary beverages, helping individuals stay hydrated without the added sugars and calories.

Precautions and Considerations:

Consultation: Individuals with certain medical conditions or allergies should consult with a healthcare provider before incorporating Gymnema Sylvestre tea into their diet, especially if they are taking medications or supplements.

Monitoring: Regular monitoring of blood sugar levels is essential, allowing individuals to assess the effects of Gymnema Sylvestre tea on blood sugar regulation and adjust consumption as needed.

Gymnema Sylvestre tea offers a flavorful and healthful beverage option for individuals managing diabetes. With its potential benefits for blood sugar regulation, reduced sugar cravings, and weight management, Gymnema Sylvestre tea can be a valuable addition to a diabetes management plan. By incorporating Gymnema Sylvestre tea into their daily routines, individuals can enjoy its delightful flavor and potential health benefits while supporting their overall health and well-being.

Fenugreek and Cinnamon Blend

Combining the aromatic flavors and potent health benefits of fenugreek and cinnamon, this diabetes tea blend offers a delicious and effective way to support blood sugar control and overall well-being. Fenugreek and cinnamon have long been used in traditional medicine for their ability to regulate blood sugar levels, making them valuable ingredients in managing diabetes.

Health Benefits of Fenugreek and Cinnamon:

Blood Sugar Regulation: Both fenugreek and cinnamon have been shown to improve insulin sensitivity and lower blood sugar levels, making them effective natural remedies for individuals with diabetes.

Antioxidant Properties: Fenugreek and cinnamon are rich in antioxidants, which help combat oxidative stress and inflammation in the body, supporting overall health and well-being.

Digestive Health: Fenugreek contains soluble fiber, which aids in digestion and may help regulate blood sugar levels. Cinnamon also supports digestive health by reducing bloating and improving gut motility.

Impact on Blood Sugar Regulation:
The combination of fenugreek and cinnamon in this tea blend provides synergistic effects, enhancing their individual benefits for blood sugar control. Fenugreek helps improve insulin sensitivity and reduce sugar absorption, while cinnamon enhances glucose metabolism and insulin sensitivity, resulting in better blood sugar regulation.

Flavor Profile and Preparation:

Warm and Spicy: The combination of fenugreek and cinnamon creates a warm and spicy flavor profile with earthy undertones, providing a comforting and satisfying drinking experience.

Preparation: To prepare the fenugreek and cinnamon blend tea, combine dried fenugreek seeds or leaves with cinnamon sticks in hot water. Allow the mixture to steep for 10-15 minutes to infuse fully. Strain and serve plain or with a touch of honey for sweetness, if desired.

Incorporating Fenugreek and Cinnamon Blend into a Diabetes Management Plan:

Regular Consumption: Enjoying the fenugreek and cinnamon blend tea as part of a balanced diet and lifestyle can provide a flavorful and healthful way to support blood sugar control and overall well-being.

Hydration Alternative: The fenugreek and cinnamon blend tea can serve as a hydrating alternative to sugary beverages, helping individuals stay hydrated without the added sugars and calories.

Precautions and Considerations:

Consultation: Individuals with certain medical conditions or allergies should consult with a healthcare provider before incorporating the fenugreek and cinnamon blend tea into their diet, especially if they are taking medications or supplements.

Monitoring: Regular monitoring of blood sugar levels is essential, allowing individuals to assess the effects of the fenugreek and cinnamon blend tea on blood sugar regulation and adjust consumption as needed.

The fenugreek and cinnamon blend tea offers a flavorful and healthful beverage option for individuals managing diabetes. With its combined benefits for blood sugar regulation, antioxidant properties, and digestive health, this tea blend can be a valuable addition to a diabetes management plan. By incorporating the fenugreek and cinnamon blend tea into their daily routines, individuals can enjoy its delightful flavor and potential health benefits while supporting their overall health and well-being.

CHAPTER EIGHT

Diabetic neuropathy is a common complication of diabetes that affects the nerves, often leading to symptoms such as numbness, tingling, and pain in the extremities. While medical treatments are available, incorporating healing teas into a diabetes management plan can provide additional support for managing neuropathy symptoms and reducing the risk of complications. This comprehensive guide explores various healing teas that may benefit individuals with diabetic neuropathy and associated complications.

1. Chamomile Tea:

Benefits: Chamomile tea possesses anti-inflammatory and antioxidant properties, which may help reduce inflammation and oxidative stress associated with diabetic neuropathy. Additionally, chamomile's calming effects can promote relaxation and alleviate stress, potentially improving neuropathy symptoms.

2. **Ginger Tea:**

Benefits: Ginger tea has analgesic and anti-inflammatory properties, making it effective for relieving neuropathic pain and inflammation. Moreover, ginger can help improve circulation, which is essential for preventing and managing diabetic neuropathy.

3. **Turmeric Tea:**

Benefits: Turmeric contains curcumin, a compound with potent anti-inflammatory and antioxidant properties. Drinking turmeric tea may help reduce inflammation and oxidative stress, thereby alleviating neuropathy symptoms and promoting nerve health.

4. **Green Tea:**

Benefits: Green tea is rich in polyphenols and antioxidants, which have neuroprotective effects and may help prevent or delay the progression of diabetic neuropathy. Regular consumption of green tea can also improve blood circulation and support overall nerve health.

5. Lemon Balm Tea:

Benefits: Lemon balm tea has soothing properties that can help relieve neuropathic pain and discomfort. Additionally, lemon balm may improve sleep quality and reduce stress levels, which are important factors in managing neuropathy symptoms.

6. Holy Basil Tea:

Benefits: Holy basil, or Tulsi, has adaptogenic properties that can help the body cope with stress and reduce inflammation. Drinking holy basil tea may alleviate neuropathic pain and improve overall nerve function.

7. Cinnamon Tea:

Benefits: Cinnamon has been shown to improve blood sugar control and reduce inflammation, making it beneficial for individuals with diabetic neuropathy. Regular consumption of cinnamon tea may help alleviate neuropathic symptoms and prevent further nerve damage.

8. **Fenugreek Tea:**
Benefits: Fenugreek contains compounds that can help regulate blood sugar levels and reduce inflammation. Drinking fenugreek tea may help improve nerve function and alleviate neuropathic pain associated with diabetes.

Incorporating Healing Teas into a Diabetes Management Plan:

Regular Consumption: Drink healing teas regularly as part of a balanced diet and lifestyle to reap their benefits for managing diabetic neuropathy and complications.

Hydration: Use healing teas as a hydrating alternative to sugary beverages, promoting overall health and well-being while supporting nerve health.

Precautions and Considerations:

Consultation: Individuals with diabetes should consult with a healthcare provider before incorporating healing teas into their diet, especially if they are taking medications or supplements.

Monitoring: Regular monitoring of blood sugar levels and neuropathy symptoms is essential to assess the effects of healing teas and adjust consumption as needed.

Incorporating healing teas into a diabetes management plan can provide valuable support for individuals with diabetic neuropathy and associated complications. By including these teas in their daily routine, individuals can harness their beneficial properties to alleviate symptoms, promote nerve health, and enhance overall well-being. With their natural healing properties and soothing effects, healing teas offer a comforting and effective approach to managing diabetic neuropathy and complications.

Chamomile Tea

Chamomile tea, derived from the dried flowers of the chamomile plant, is renowned for its soothing properties and pleasant aroma. Beyond its calming effects, chamomile tea offers potential benefits for individuals managing diabetes. With its anti-inflammatory and antioxidant properties, chamomile tea can be a valuable addition to a diabetes-friendly diet and lifestyle.

Health Benefits of Chamomile Tea:

Blood Sugar Regulation: Chamomile tea may help regulate blood sugar levels by improving insulin sensitivity and reducing inflammation in the body. Regular consumption of chamomile tea has been associated with improved glycemic control in individuals with diabetes.

Stress Reduction: Stress can adversely affect blood sugar levels and exacerbate diabetes symptoms. Chamomile tea's calming effects can help reduce stress and promote relaxation, which is beneficial for overall diabetes management.

Digestive Health: Chamomile tea has been traditionally used to alleviate digestive issues such as indigestion, bloating, and gas. A healthy digestive system is essential for optimal nutrient absorption and blood sugar regulation.

Impact on Blood Sugar Regulation: Research suggests that chamomile tea may help improve insulin sensitivity and reduce blood sugar levels, making it a valuable beverage for individuals with diabetes. By incorporating chamomile tea into their daily routine, individuals may experience better blood sugar control and overall well-being.

Flavor Profile and Preparation:

Mild and Floral: Chamomile tea has a mild and slightly floral flavor profile, with subtle hints of apple and sweetness. It is soothing and comforting, making it an ideal beverage for relaxation.

Preparation: To prepare chamomile tea, steep dried chamomile flowers in hot water for 5-10 minutes, allowing the flavors to infuse fully. Strain and serve plain or with a touch of honey for sweetness, if desired.

Incorporating Chamomile Tea into a Diabetes Management Plan:

Regular Consumption: Enjoying chamomile tea as part of a balanced diet and lifestyle can provide a flavorful and healthful way to support blood sugar control and reduce stress levels.

Hydration Alternative: Chamomile tea can serve as a hydrating alternative to sugary beverages, helping individuals stay hydrated without the added sugars and calories.

Precautions and Considerations:

Consultation: Individuals with certain medical conditions or allergies should consult with a healthcare provider before incorporating chamomile tea into their diet, especially if they are taking medications or supplements.

Monitoring: Regular monitoring of blood sugar levels is essential, allowing individuals to assess the effects of chamomile tea on blood sugar regulation and adjust consumption as needed.

Chamomile tea offers a flavorful and healthful beverage option for individuals managing diabetes. With its potential benefits for blood sugar regulation, stress reduction, and digestive health, chamomile tea can be a valuable addition to a diabetes management plan. By incorporating chamomile tea into their daily routines, individuals can enjoy its delightful flavor and potential health benefits while supporting their overall health and well-being.

Lavender Tea

Lavender tea, made from the dried flowers of the lavender plant, is celebrated for its delightful aroma and calming properties. While primarily known for its relaxation benefits, lavender tea also offers potential advantages for individuals managing diabetes. With its anti-inflammatory and antioxidant properties, lavender tea can be a soothing addition to a diabetes-friendly diet and lifestyle.

Health Benefits of Lavender Tea:

Blood Sugar Regulation: Lavender tea may help regulate blood sugar levels by reducing inflammation and oxidative stress in the body. Studies suggest that lavender extract may improve insulin sensitivity and glucose metabolism, which are crucial factors in diabetes management.

Stress Reduction: Stress can negatively impact blood sugar control and exacerbate diabetes symptoms. Lavender tea's calming effects can help reduce stress and promote relaxation, contributing to better overall diabetes management.

Sleep Support: Lavender tea is renowned for its ability to promote restful sleep and alleviate insomnia symptoms. Quality sleep is essential for regulating blood sugar levels and supporting overall health, making lavender tea a beneficial beverage for individuals with diabetes.

Impact on Blood Sugar Regulation:
While research specifically on lavender tea's effects on blood sugar regulation is limited, the anti-inflammatory and antioxidant properties of lavender may indirectly benefit individuals with diabetes. By promoting overall health and reducing stress levels, lavender tea can support better blood sugar control and diabetes management.

Flavor Profile and Preparation:

Subtle and Floral: Lavender tea has a subtle and floral flavor profile, with hints of sweetness and herbaceousness. It is gentle and calming, making it a soothing beverage choice.

Preparation: To prepare lavender tea, steep dried lavender flowers in hot water for 5-10 minutes, allowing the flavors to infuse fully. Strain and serve plain or with a touch of honey for sweetness, if desired.

Incorporating Lavender Tea into a Diabetes Management Plan:

Regular Consumption: Enjoying lavender tea as part of a balanced diet and lifestyle can provide a flavorful and healthful way to support blood sugar control and reduce stress levels.

Evening Ritual: Drinking lavender tea in the evening can promote relaxation and improve sleep quality, leading to better blood sugar regulation and overall well-being.

Precautions and Considerations:

Consultation: Individuals with certain medical conditions or allergies should consult with a healthcare provider before incorporating lavender tea into their diet, especially if they are taking medications or supplements.

Moderation: While lavender tea is generally safe for most people, excessive consumption may cause adverse effects. It is recommended to drink lavender tea in moderation as part of a varied diet.

Lavender tea offers a flavorful and healthful beverage option for individuals managing diabetes. With its potential benefits for blood sugar regulation, stress reduction, and sleep support, lavender tea can be a valuable addition to a diabetes management plan. By incorporating lavender tea into their daily routines, individuals can enjoy its delightful flavor and potential health benefits while supporting their overall health and well-being.

Lemon Balm Tea

Lemon balm tea, crafted from the leaves of the lemon balm plant, is cherished for its refreshing citrus flavor and calming properties. While often enjoyed for its soothing effects on the mind and body, lemon balm tea also offers potential benefits for individuals managing diabetes. With its anti-inflammatory and antioxidant properties, lemon balm tea can be a flavorful addition to a diabetes-friendly diet and lifestyle.

Health Benefits of Lemon Balm Tea:

Blood Sugar Regulation: Lemon balm tea may help regulate blood sugar levels by reducing inflammation and oxidative stress in the body. Studies suggest that lemon balm extract may improve insulin sensitivity and glucose metabolism, contributing to better blood sugar control.

Stress Reduction: Stress can adversely affect blood sugar levels and exacerbate diabetes symptoms. Lemon balm tea's calming effects can help reduce stress and promote relaxation, supporting overall diabetes management.

Digestive Health: Lemon balm tea has been traditionally used to alleviate digestive issues such as indigestion, bloating, and gas. A healthy digestive system is essential for optimal nutrient absorption and blood sugar regulation.

Impact on Blood Sugar Regulation:

While research specifically on lemon balm tea's effects on blood sugar regulation is limited, its anti-inflammatory and antioxidant properties may indirectly benefit individuals with diabetes. By promoting overall health and reducing stress levels, lemon balm tea can support better blood sugar control and diabetes management.

Flavor Profile and Preparation:

Citrusy and Refreshing: Lemon balm tea has a bright and citrusy flavor profile, with subtle herbal undertones. It is uplifting and invigorating, making it a delightful beverage choice.

Preparation: To prepare lemon balm tea, steep dried lemon balm leaves in hot water for 5-10 minutes, allowing the flavors to infuse fully. Strain and serve plain or with a slice of lemon for extra citrus flavor, if desired.

Incorporating Lemon Balm Tea into a Diabetes Management Plan:

Regular Consumption: Enjoying lemon balm tea as part of a balanced diet and lifestyle can provide a flavorful and healthful way to support blood sugar control and reduce stress levels.

Hydration Alternative: Lemon balm tea can serve as a hydrating alternative to sugary beverages, helping individuals stay hydrated without the added sugars and calories.

Precautions and Considerations:

Consultation: Individuals with certain medical conditions or allergies should consult with a healthcare provider before incorporating lemon balm tea into their diet, especially if they are taking medications or supplements.

Moderation: While lemon balm tea is generally safe for most people, excessive consumption may cause adverse effects. It is recommended to drink lemon balm tea in moderation as part of a varied diet.

Passionflower Tea

Passionflower tea, derived from the dried leaves and flowers of the passion flower plant, is esteemed for its calming and sedative properties. While primarily known for its ability to promote relaxation and alleviate anxiety, passionflower tea also offers potential benefits for individuals managing diabetes. With its anti-inflammatory and antioxidant properties, passionflower tea can be a soothing addition to a diabetes-friendly diet and lifestyle.

Health Benefits of Passionflower Tea:

Blood Sugar Regulation: Passionflower tea may help regulate blood sugar levels by reducing inflammation and oxidative stress in the body. Studies suggest that passionflower extract may improve insulin sensitivity and glucose metabolism, contributing to better blood sugar control.

Stress Reduction: Stress can negatively impact blood sugar control and exacerbate diabetes symptoms. Passionflower tea's calming effects can help reduce stress and promote relaxation, supporting overall diabetes management.

Sleep Support: Passionflower tea is renowned for its ability to improve sleep quality and duration. Quality sleep is essential for regulating blood sugar levels and supporting overall health, making passionflower tea a beneficial beverage for individuals with diabetes.

Impact on Blood Sugar Regulation:
While research specifically on passion flower tea's effects on blood sugar regulation is limited, its anti-inflammatory and antioxidant properties may indirectly benefit individuals with diabetes. By promoting overall health and reducing stress levels, passionflower tea can support better blood sugar control and diabetes management.

Flavor Profile and Preparation:

Subtle and Floral: Passionflower tea has a subtle and floral flavor profile, with hints of sweetness and herbaceousness. It is gentle and calming, making it an ideal beverage for relaxation.

Preparation: To prepare passionflower tea, steep dried passion flower leaves and flowers in hot water for 5-10 minutes, allowing the flavors to infuse fully. Strain and serve plain or with a touch of honey for sweetness, if desired.

Incorporating Passionflower Tea into a Diabetes Management Plan:

Regular Consumption: Enjoying passionflower tea as part of a balanced diet and lifestyle can provide a flavorful and healthful way to support blood sugar control and reduce stress levels.

Evening Ritual: Drinking passionflower tea in the evening can promote relaxation and improve sleep quality, leading to better blood sugar regulation and overall well-being.

Precautions and Considerations:

Consultation: Individuals with certain medical conditions or allergies should consult with a healthcare provider before incorporating passionflower tea into their diet, especially if they are taking medications or supplements.

Moderation: While passionflower tea is generally safe for most people, excessive consumption may cause adverse effects. It is recommended to drink passionflower tea in moderation as part of a varied diet.

Valerian Root Tea

Valerian root tea, brewed from the dried roots of the Valeriana plant, is esteemed for its calming and sedative properties. While primarily known for its ability to promote relaxation and alleviate insomnia, valerian root tea also offers potential benefits for Individuals managing diabetes. With its anti-inflammatory and antioxidant properties, valerian root tea can be a soothing addition to a diabetes-friendly diet and lifestyle.

Health Benefits of Valerian Root Tea:

Blood Sugar Regulation: Valerian root tea may help regulate blood sugar levels by reducing inflammation and oxidative stress in the body. Studies suggest that valerian extract may improve insulin sensitivity and glucose metabolism, contributing to better blood sugar control.

Stress Reduction: Stress can negatively impact blood sugar control and exacerbate diabetes symptoms. Valerian root tea's calming effects can help reduce stress and promote relaxation, supporting overall diabetes management.

Sleep Support: Valerian root tea is renowned for its ability to improve sleep quality and duration. Quality sleep is essential for regulating blood sugar levels and supporting overall health, making valerian root tea a beneficial beverage for individuals with diabetes.

Impact on Blood Sugar Regulation: While research specifically on valerian root tea's effects on blood sugar regulation is limited, its anti-inflammatory and antioxidant properties may indirectly benefit individuals with diabetes. By promoting overall health and reducing stress levels, valerian root tea can support better blood sugar control and diabetes management.

Flavor Profile and Preparation:

Earthy and Pungent: Valerian root tea has an earthy and slightly pungent flavor profile, with herbal undertones. It is grounding and soothing, making it an ideal beverage for relaxation.

Preparation: To prepare valerian root tea, steep dried valerian roots in hot water for 5-10 minutes, allowing the flavors to infuse fully. Strain and serve plain or with a touch of honey for sweetness, if desired.

Incorporating Valerian Root Tea into a Diabetes Management Plan:

Regular Consumption: Enjoying valerian root tea as part of a balanced diet and lifestyle can provide a flavorful and healthful way to support blood sugar control and reduce stress levels.

Evening Ritual: Drinking valerian root tea in the evening can promote relaxation and improve sleep quality, leading to better blood sugar regulation and overall well-being.

Precautions and Considerations:

Consultation: Individuals with certain medical conditions or allergies should consult with a healthcare provider before incorporating valerian root tea into their diet, especially if they are taking medications or supplements.

Moderation: While valerian root tea is generally safe for most people, excessive consumption may cause adverse effects. It is recommended to drink valerian root tea in moderation as part of a varied diet.

Valerian root tea offers a flavorful and healthful beverage option for individuals managing diabetes. With its potential benefits for blood sugar regulation, stress reduction, and sleep support, valerian root tea can be a valuable addition to a diabetes management plan. By incorporating valerian root tea into their daily routines, individuals can enjoy its delightful flavor and potential health benefits while supporting their overall health and well-being.

CHAPTER NINE

Tea Rituals and Lifestyle Changes for Diabetes Wellness

Incorporating tea rituals into daily life can be a soothing and healthful practice, especially for individuals managing diabetes. Tea, particularly herbal teas, offers a variety of potential benefits for diabetes management, including blood sugar regulation, stress reduction, and hydration. By combining tea rituals with lifestyle changes, individuals can enhance their overall wellness and better manage their diabetes.

Tea Rituals for Diabetes Wellness:

Morning Ritual: Start the day with a calming cup of herbal tea, such as chamomile or ginger tea. These teas can help reduce morning stress and promote relaxation, setting a positive tone for the day ahead.

Afternoon Pick-Me-Up: Enjoy a refreshing cup of green tea or lemon balm tea in the afternoon to boost energy levels and improve focus. These teas can also help regulate blood sugar levels and curb cravings for unhealthy snacks.

Evening Wind-Down: Wind down in the evening with a soothing cup of lavender or passionflower tea. These teas can promote relaxation and improve sleep quality, essential for overall wellness and blood sugar control.

Lifestyle Changes for Diabetes Wellness:

Healthy Eating: Focus on a balanced diet rich in whole foods, fruits, vegetables, lean proteins, and healthy fats. Limit intake of processed foods, sugary snacks, and high-carbohydrate meals to help manage blood sugar levels.

Regular Exercise: Incorporate regular physical activity into your daily routine, such as walking, cycling, or yoga. Exercise helps improve insulin sensitivity, regulate blood sugar levels, and promote overall well-being.

Stress Management: Practice stress-reducing techniques such as meditation, deep breathing exercises, or mindfulness practices. Chronic stress can negatively impact blood sugar control, so finding healthy ways to manage stress is crucial for diabetes wellness.

Hydration: Stay hydrated throughout the day by drinking plenty of water and herbal teas. Hydration is essential for overall health and can help regulate blood sugar levels.

Incorporating Tea Rituals into Lifestyle Changes:

Mindful Consumption: Practice mindfulness while drinking tea, savoring each sip and taking time to appreciate the flavors and aromas. This mindful approach can extend to other aspects of life, promoting overall well-being.

Social Connection: Enjoying tea with friends and family can foster social connection and provide support in managing diabetes. Host tea parties or gatherings where herbal teas are served alongside healthy snacks and conversation.

Tea rituals and lifestyle changes can play a significant role in promoting wellness for individuals managing diabetes. By incorporating herbal teas into daily routines and making healthy lifestyle choices, individuals can improve blood sugar control, reduce stress levels, and enhance overall well-being.

Mindful Tea Drinking Practices

Mindful tea drinking involves being fully present and attentive while enjoying a cup of tea. This practice can have numerous benefits for individuals managing diabetes, including stress reduction, blood sugar regulation, and overall well-being. By incorporating mindful tea drinking practices into daily life, individuals can cultivate a deeper connection with their tea experience and support their diabetes management goals.

Benefits of Mindful Tea Drinking:

Stress Reduction: Mindful tea drinking encourages relaxation and stress reduction by focusing attention on the present moment. This can help alleviate stress, which is beneficial for blood sugar control and overall health.

Blood Sugar Regulation: Mindful tea drinking promotes mindful eating habits, which can help regulate blood sugar levels. By paying attention to hunger cues and enjoying tea without distractions, individuals can better manage their blood sugar levels.

Enhanced Enjoyment: Mindful tea drinking allows individuals to fully appreciate the flavors, aromas, and textures of their tea. This can enhance the enjoyment of the tea-drinking experience and promote a sense of well-being.

Mindful Tea Drinking Practices:

Set the Scene: Create a peaceful environment for tea drinking by choosing a quiet and comfortable space free from distractions. Settle into a cozy chair or find a tranquil spot in nature to enjoy your tea.

Engage the Senses: Before taking a sip, take a moment to engage your senses. Notice the aroma of the tea as it steeps, the warmth of the cup in your hands, and the color of the tea as you pour it into your cup.

Savor Each Sip: Take small, mindful sips of your tea, allowing the flavors to linger on your palate. Pay attention to the taste, texture, and temperature of the tea as you drink it.

Practice Gratitude: As you enjoy your tea, take a moment to express gratitude for the experience. Reflect on the journey of the tea from plant to cup and appreciate the nourishment it provides for your body and soul.

Be Present: Let go of distractions and worries, and focus your attention fully on the present moment. Notice any thoughts or emotions that arise without judgment, and gently bring your focus back to the sensations of tea drinking.

Incorporating Mindful Tea Drinking into Diabetes Management:

Stress Management: Mindful tea drinking can be a valuable tool for managing stress, which is closely linked to diabetes management. By practicing mindfulness while drinking tea, individuals can reduce stress levels and support better blood sugar control.

Healthy Eating Habits: Mindful tea drinking encourages mindful eating habits, such as paying attention to hunger cues and enjoying food and beverages without distractions. This can support healthy eating habits and blood sugar regulation.

Mindful tea drinking is a simple yet powerful practice that can benefit individuals managing diabetes. By cultivating mindfulness while enjoying a cup of tea, individuals can reduce stress, regulate blood sugar levels, and enhance their overall well-being.

Stress Management Techniques

Stress management is essential for individuals managing diabetes, as stress can negatively impact blood sugar levels and overall health. Incorporating stress management techniques into daily life can help individuals cope with stressors more effectively and support their diabetes management goals. Alongside enjoying diabetes-friendly teas, practicing stress management techniques can promote a sense of calm and well-being.

Stress Management Techniques:

Mindfulness Meditation: Mindfulness meditation is concentrating on the here and now while impartially examining one's thoughts and emotions. Frequent practice can improve both physical and mental health by lowering stress levels and encouraging relaxation.

Deep Breathing Exercises: Deep breathing techniques, like belly breathing and diaphragmatic breathing, can help lower tension and trigger the body's relaxation response. Breathing deeply and slowly can help to develop calmness and peace of mind by calming the nervous system.

Progressive Muscle Relaxation: Progressive muscle relaxation involves tensing and then relaxing different muscle groups in the body, systematically releasing tension and promoting relaxation. This technique can help individuals become more aware of muscle tension and learn to let go of stress.

Yoga and Tai Chi: Yoga and Tai Chi are gentle forms of exercise that combine physical postures, breathing techniques, and meditation. These practices can help reduce stress, improve flexibility and balance, and promote overall well-being.

Journaling: Writing in a journal can be a therapeutic way to express thoughts and feelings, identify sources of stress, and develop coping strategies. Regular journaling can help individuals gain insight into their emotions and reduce stress levels.

Spending Time in Nature: Spending time outdoors in nature can have a calming effect on the mind and body. Activities such as walking, hiking, or gardening can help reduce stress and promote relaxation.

Incorporating Tea Rituals into Stress Management:

Mindful Tea Drinking: Engaging in mindful tea drinking practices can enhance the stress-relieving benefits of tea. By savoring each sip and focusing on the present moment, individuals can promote relaxation and reduce stress levels.

Herbal Teas for Stress Relief: Certain herbal teas, such as chamomile, lavender, and lemon balm, are known for their calming properties and can be incorporated into a stress management routine. Enjoying a cup of herbal tea can help promote relaxation and reduce stress after a long day.

Managing stress is an important aspect of diabetes management, as stress can impact blood sugar levels and overall well-being. By incorporating stress management techniques into daily life, individuals can better cope with stressors and support their diabetes management goals. Alongside practicing mindfulness, deep breathing exercises, and other stress management techniques, individuals can enjoy diabetes-friendly teas as part of a soothing and healthful stress management routine.

Sleep Hygiene Tips

Quality sleep is essential for overall health and well-being, especially for individuals managing diabetes. Poor sleep can negatively impact blood sugar control, energy levels, and overall health. Practicing good sleep hygiene can help improve sleep quality and promote better diabetes management. Alongside enjoying diabetes-friendly teas, implementing sleep hygiene tips can support a restful night's sleep.

Sleep Hygiene Tips:

Keep a Regular Sleep Schedule: Even on weekends, go to bed and wake up at the same time every day. Maintaining consistency improves the quality of sleep and aids the body's internal clock.

Establish a Calm nighttime ritual: To let your body know when it's time to wind down, create a calm nighttime ritual. This could involve reading, having a warm bath, or engaging in relaxation exercises like meditation or deep breathing.

Optimize Your Sleep Environment: Create a sleep-friendly environment that is cool, dark, and quiet. Use blackout curtains or a sleep mask to block out light, and consider using earplugs or a white noise machine to mask any disruptive sounds.

Limit Screen Time Before Bed: At least one hour before going to bed, limit your time spent in front of screens, including computers, tablets, and cellphones. Screen blue light can interfere with melatonin production and cause sleep patterns to be disturbed.

Watch Your Caffeine Intake: Limit caffeine intake, especially in the afternoon and evening, as it can interfere with sleep. Opt for caffeine-free herbal teas, such as chamomile or lavender, in the evening to promote relaxation.

Manage Stress: Practice stress management techniques, such as deep breathing exercises, meditation, or yoga, to help calm the mind and body before bedtime. Managing stress can promote relaxation and improve sleep quality.

Limit Alcohol and Large Meals Before Bed: These two things might cause sleep disturbances and restless nights. So, steer clear of them just before bed. If you're hungry right before bed, choose light, simple-to-digest foods.

Exercise Frequently: Get moving on a regular basis, but steer clear of strenuous exercise right before bed. Exercise can support improved general wellbeing and the quality of sleep.

Incorporating Tea Rituals into Sleep Hygiene:

Bedtime Tea Ritual: Enjoying a cup of caffeine-free herbal tea, such as chamomile or valerian root, as part of your bedtime routine can promote relaxation and signal to your body that it's time to wind down.

Relaxing Tea Blends: Experiment with different herbal tea blends known for their calming properties, such as lavender, passionflower, or lemon balm, to find the perfect bedtime brew that promotes relaxation and supports restful sleep.

Practicing good sleep hygiene is essential for individuals managing diabetes to promote better blood sugar control and overall health. By incorporating sleep hygiene tips into your daily routine and enjoying diabetes-friendly teas as part of a soothing bedtime ritual, you can improve sleep quality and support your diabetes management goals. Prioritizing sleep hygiene can lead to more restful nights and improved well-being overall.

Incorporating Tea into a Balanced Lifestyle

Tea is more than just a beverage; it's a versatile and healthful addition to a balanced lifestyle, especially for individuals managing diabetes. With a wide variety of flavors and health benefits, tea can be enjoyed throughout the day as part of a diabetes-friendly diet and lifestyle. By incorporating tea into your daily routine, you can promote hydration, support blood sugar control, and enhance overall well-being.

Benefits of Tea in a Balanced Lifestyle:

Hydration: Tea can help you meet your daily fluid intake requirements. Staying hydrated is important for your general health. Drinking a range of herbal teas, such hibiscus, peppermint, or chamomile, can help you stay hydrated all day.

Blood Sugar Regulation: Certain types of tea, such as green tea and herbal teas, have been shown to support blood sugar control. By incorporating these teas into your daily routine, you can help regulate blood sugar levels and support your diabetes management goals.

Antioxidant Support: Tea is rich in antioxidants, which help protect cells from damage caused by free radicals. Antioxidants have been linked to a reduced risk of chronic diseases, including diabetes, making tea a valuable addition to a balanced lifestyle.

Stress Reduction: Enjoying a soothing cup of tea can help promote relaxation and reduce stress levels. Herbal teas like chamomile, lavender, and passionflower are particularly known for their calming properties, making them ideal choices for stress relief.

Variety and Flavor: With countless varieties and flavors to choose from, tea offers endless possibilities for enjoyment. Whether you prefer classic green tea, spicy chai, or fragrant herbal blends, there's a tea to suit every taste preference and mood.

Incorporating Tea into Your Daily Routine:

Morning Boost: Start your day with a refreshing cup of green tea or herbal tea to kickstart your morning and hydrate your body. Experiment with different flavors and blends to find your favorite morning brew.

Midday Pick-Me-Up: Enjoy a midday break with a cup of herbal tea or a revitalizing iced tea. Herbal teas like peppermint or ginger can help refresh your senses and provide a natural energy boost without caffeine.

Evening Relaxation: Wind down in the evening with a soothing cup of chamomile, lavender, or valerian root tea. These herbal teas can help promote relaxation and prepare your body and mind for a restful night's sleep.

Social Gatherings: Incorporate tea into social gatherings by hosting tea parties or afternoon tea sessions with friends and family. Explore different tea varieties and share the joy of tea together.

Incorporating tea into a balanced lifestyle can provide numerous benefits for individuals managing diabetes. From supporting hydration and blood sugar control to promoting relaxation and enjoyment, tea offers a wealth of possibilities for enhancing overall well-being. By incorporating tea into your daily routine and exploring the diverse world of tea, you can cultivate a healthier and more balanced lifestyle while managing your diabetes effectively.

CHAPTER TEN

Holistic Approaches: Mindfulness, Meditation, and Tea for Diabetes

Holistic approaches that encompass mindfulness, meditation, and the incorporation of tea into daily life can offer valuable support for individuals managing diabetes. These practices focus on nurturing the mind, body, and spirit, promoting overall well-being and aiding in diabetes management. By integrating mindfulness, meditation, and tea rituals into their routine, individuals can cultivate a holistic approach to diabetes care that addresses both physical and emotional needs.

Mindfulness for Diabetes Management:

Awareness of Body and Sensations:
Mindfulness involves paying attention to the
present moment with openness and curiosity.
By tuning into bodily sensations, such as
hunger cues and blood sugar fluctuations,
individuals can make informed choices that
support their diabetes management goals.

Managing Stress and Emotions: Mindfulness
practices help individuals recognize and
manage stress and emotional responses
associated with diabetes. By developing a
non-judgmental awareness of thoughts and
feelings, individuals can cultivate resilience and
cope more effectively with the challenges of
living with diabetes.

Meditation for Diabetes Management:

Stress Reduction: Meditation techniques, such as focused breathing or body scan meditation, can promote relaxation and reduce stress levels. Chronic stress can adversely affect blood sugar levels, so incorporating meditation into daily life can have positive effects on diabetes management.

Improved Blood Sugar Control: Some studies suggest that regular meditation practice may improve blood sugar control and insulin sensitivity in individuals with diabetes. By reducing stress hormones and promoting a state of relaxation, meditation may help regulate blood sugar levels more effectively.

Incorporating Tea Rituals into Holistic Diabetes Care:

Mindful Tea Drinking: Tea rituals provide an opportunity for mindful engagement with the senses, promoting relaxation and stress reduction. By savoring each sip of tea, individuals can cultivate mindfulness and enhance their overall well-being.

Herbal Teas for Health: Herbal teas, such as chamomile, ginger, or cinnamon tea, offer a variety of health benefits that can support diabetes management. Whether it's promoting relaxation, aiding digestion, or improving blood sugar control, herbal teas can be a valuable addition to a holistic diabetes care regimen.

Practical Tips for Integration:

Daily Practice: Incorporate mindfulness meditation into your daily routine, setting aside dedicated time each day for practice. Likewise, make tea drinking a mindful ritual by pausing to appreciate the flavors and aromas of your tea.

Community Support: Joining a meditation group or tea club can provide social support and accountability, enhancing the effectiveness of these practices for diabetes management.

Holistic approaches encompassing mindfulness, meditation, and the incorporation of tea into daily life offer valuable support for individuals managing diabetes. By cultivating mindfulness, reducing stress, and embracing tea rituals, individuals can promote overall well-being and enhance their diabetes management efforts.

The Connection Between Mind-Body Practices and Blood Sugar Regulation

The relationship between mind-body practices, such as mindfulness, meditation, and yoga, and blood sugar regulation is a topic of growing interest in diabetes management. These holistic approaches focus on nurturing the connection between the mind and body, promoting overall well-being, and potentially impacting blood sugar levels in individuals with diabetes. By incorporating mind-body practices alongside diabetes-friendly teas, individuals can support their blood sugar regulation efforts and enhance their overall health.

**Mind-Body Practices for Blood Sugar
Regulation:**

Stress Reduction: Mind-body practices are
known for their ability to reduce stress levels,
which is particularly beneficial for individuals
managing diabetes. Chronic stress can elevate
blood sugar levels through the release of
stress hormones like cortisol, so reducing
stress can help promote better blood sugar
control.

Improving Insulin Sensitivity: Some research
suggests that mind-body practices, such as
meditation and yoga, may improve insulin
sensitivity in individuals with diabetes. By
reducing stress and promoting relaxation,
these practices can enhance the body's ability
to respond to insulin and regulate blood sugar
levels more effectively.

Enhancing Mindfulness: Mindfulness practices cultivate awareness of the present moment and encourage non-judgmental acceptance of thoughts and feelings. By incorporating mindfulness into daily life, individuals can develop a deeper understanding of their body's signals, including hunger cues and blood sugar fluctuations, and make healthier choices to support blood sugar regulation.

The Role of Tea in Mind-Body Practices:

Mindful Tea Drinking: Enjoying a cup of tea mindfully can complement mind-body practices by promoting relaxation and enhancing the overall sensory experience. By savoring each sip of tea and paying attention to the flavors and aromas, individuals can cultivate mindfulness and support their blood sugar regulation efforts.

Herbal Teas for Relaxation: Certain herbal teas, such as chamomile, lavender, and lemon balm, are renowned for their calming properties and can be incorporated into mind-body practices to promote relaxation and stress reduction. These teas can be enjoyed before or after meditation or yoga sessions to enhance the overall experience.

Practical Tips for Integration:

Consistent Practice: Incorporate mind-body practices into your daily routine, setting aside dedicated time each day for meditation, mindfulness, or yoga. Likewise, make tea drinking a regular part of your routine, choosing diabetes-friendly herbal teas to support relaxation and stress reduction.

Mindful Eating: Practice mindful eating alongside mind-body practices and tea drinking, paying attention to hunger cues and enjoying your meals without distractions. Mindful eating can help regulate food intake and support blood sugar regulation.

The connection between mind-body practices
and blood sugar regulation underscores the
importance of holistic approaches in diabetes
management. By incorporating mindfulness,
meditation, yoga, and tea into daily life,
individuals can support their blood sugar
regulation efforts, reduce stress levels, and
enhance their overall well-being. Through a
holistic approach that addresses both physical
and emotional aspects of health, individuals
can achieve greater balance and vitality while
managing diabetes effectively.

Meditation and Its Impact on Stress Reduction

Meditation is a powerful practice that can have profound effects on stress reduction, which is particularly beneficial for individuals managing diabetes. Chronic stress can negatively impact blood sugar levels and overall health, making stress management an essential component of diabetes care. By incorporating meditation into their daily routine alongside diabetes-friendly teas, individuals can effectively reduce stress levels and support their overall well-being.

Understanding Meditation:
Meditation is a mind-body practice that involves focusing the mind and cultivating awareness of the present moment. There are various forms of meditation, including mindfulness meditation, focused breathing meditation, and loving-kindness meditation. These practices aim to quiet the mind, reduce stress, and promote relaxation.

Impact of Meditation on Stress Reduction:
Calming the Mind: Meditation helps calm the mind and reduce the impact of stressful thoughts and emotions. By cultivating a sense of inner peace and tranquility, meditation can alleviate feelings of anxiety and overwhelm associated with chronic stress.

Regulating Stress Hormones: Meditation has been shown to reduce the production of stress hormones such as cortisol and adrenaline. By modulating the body's stress response, meditation helps lower overall stress levels and promote a sense of calmness and well-being.

Promoting Relaxation: The deep relaxation experienced during meditation can counteract the physical symptoms of stress, such as muscle tension and elevated heart rate. Regular meditation practice trains the body to enter a state of relaxation more easily, even in the face of stressful situations.

Incorporating Meditation into Daily Life:

Consistent Practice: Dedicate a specific time each day for meditation practice, whether it's in the morning upon waking, during a lunch break, or in the evening before bed. Consistency is key to reaping the benefits of meditation for stress reduction.

Mindful Tea Drinking: Enjoy a cup of diabetes-friendly herbal tea, such as chamomile or lavender, before or after meditation to enhance the relaxation experience. Savor each sip mindfully, paying attention to the flavors and aromas of the tea.

Practical Tips for Meditation:

Find a Quiet Place: If you're going to meditate, pick a place that is peaceful, comfortable, and unoccupied. Establish a relaxing atmosphere by adding cozy furniture, gentle lighting, and even a calming scent from incense or essential oils.

Focus on the Breath: Use the breath as an anchor for your meditation practice. Focus on the sensation of the breath as it enters and leaves the body, allowing it to guide your attention and bring you into the present moment.

Non-Judgmental Awareness: Approach meditation with an attitude of openness and acceptance, allowing thoughts and feelings to arise without judgment. Simply observe them as they come and go, returning your focus to the breath whenever you become distracted.

Meditation is a valuable tool for stress reduction that can significantly benefit individuals managing diabetes. By incorporating meditation into their daily routine alongside diabetes-friendly teas, individuals can effectively lower stress levels, promote relaxation, and support their overall well-being. Through consistent practice and mindful engagement, meditation can become a powerful ally in managing the stress associated with diabetes, ultimately leading to improved health and quality of life.

Yoga for Diabetes Management

Yoga is a holistic practice that combines physical postures, breathing techniques, and meditation to promote overall well-being. For individuals managing diabetes, incorporating yoga into their routine can offer numerous benefits, including improved blood sugar control, reduced stress levels, and enhanced physical fitness. When paired with diabetes-friendly teas, yoga can be a valuable tool in managing the condition effectively.

Benefits of Yoga for Diabetes Management:

Improved Blood Sugar Control: Regular practice of yoga has been shown to improve blood sugar control in individuals with diabetes. The combination of physical movement, controlled breathing, and relaxation techniques helps regulate insulin sensitivity and promote glucose uptake by the muscles.

Stress Reduction: Yoga is renowned for its stress-relieving benefits, which can be particularly beneficial for individuals managing diabetes. Chronic stress can elevate blood sugar levels and contribute to insulin resistance, so reducing stress through yoga practice can help improve overall health and well-being.

Enhanced Physical Fitness: Yoga involves a combination of stretching, strength-building, and balance exercises, which can improve physical fitness and mobility. Regular practice can help individuals maintain a healthy weight, lower blood pressure, and reduce the risk of diabetes-related complications.

Incorporating Yoga into Diabetes Management:

Establish a Regular Practice: Set aside dedicated time each day or several times a week for yoga practice. Consistency is key to reaping the benefits of yoga for diabetes management.

Choose Diabetes-Friendly Poses: Certain yoga poses are particularly beneficial for individuals managing diabetes, including gentle stretches, twists, and inversions. Poses that focus on the abdomen, such as the cat-cow pose or seated forward bend, can help stimulate digestion and promote insulin sensitivity.

Pairing Yoga with Tea Rituals:

Pre-Yoga Hydration: Enjoy a cup of hydrating herbal tea, such as peppermint or hibiscus tea, before starting your yoga practice. Staying hydrated is essential for optimal performance and can enhance the benefits of your yoga session.

Post-Yoga Relaxation: After completing your yoga practice, unwind with a soothing cup of chamomile or lavender tea. These herbal teas can promote relaxation and help calm the mind and body after physical activity.

Practical Tips for Yoga Practice:

Listen to Your Body: Pay attention to your body's signals during yoga practice and modify poses as needed to accommodate any physical limitations or discomfort. Honor your body's needs and avoid pushing yourself beyond your limits.

Focus on Breath Awareness: Use controlled breathing techniques, such as deep belly breathing or ujjayi breath, to enhance the mind-body connection during yoga practice. Focusing on the breath can help calm the mind and promote relaxation.

Yoga is a powerful tool for diabetes management that offers numerous physical, mental, and emotional benefits. By incorporating yoga into their routine alongside diabetes-friendly teas, individuals can improve blood sugar control, reduce stress levels, and enhance overall well-being. Through consistent practice and mindful engagement, yoga can become an integral part of a holistic approach to managing diabetes effectively and living a healthier, more balanced life.

Creating Your Personalized Diabetes Wellness Plan

Managing diabetes effectively requires a personalized approach that addresses individual needs, preferences, and lifestyle factors. By creating a personalized diabetes wellness plan, individuals can tailor their approach to diabetes management and incorporate strategies that promote optimal health and well-being. Alongside diabetes-friendly teas, a personalized wellness plan can encompass various aspects of lifestyle, including diet, physical activity, stress management, and medical care.

Key Components of a Personalized Diabetes Wellness Plan:

Dietary Decisions: Create a balanced food plan that promotes blood sugar control and general health by working with a qualified dietitian or nutritionist.

Give special attention to nutrient-dense, entire foods including fruits, vegetables, lean meats, and whole grains. Include teas that are good for diabetics in your daily routine to stay hydrated and reap extra health advantages.

Physical Activity: Maintain a healthy weight, enhance insulin sensitivity, and strengthen your heart by getting regular exercise. Try to incorporate strength training, flexibility training, and cardiovascular activity into your routine. Select enjoyable activities that fit your level of fitness.

Stress Management: Develop stress management techniques to reduce the impact of stress on blood sugar levels and overall well-being. Explore mindfulness, meditation, yoga, deep breathing exercises, and other relaxation techniques to help you cope with stress more effectively.

Pair stress management practices with calming herbal teas to enhance relaxation and promote inner peace.

Blood Sugar Monitoring: Monitor blood sugar levels regularly to track your progress and make informed decisions about your diabetes management plan. Work with your healthcare team to establish target blood sugar ranges and adjust your treatment plan as needed based on your monitoring results.

Medication Management: Take medications as prescribed by your healthcare provider and follow their recommendations for insulin or other diabetes medications. Stay informed about potential side effects and interactions with other medications or supplements.

Consider incorporating herbal teas known for their potential benefits in diabetes management, but always consult with your healthcare provider before making any changes to your medication regimen.

Regular Medical Check-Ups: Schedule regular appointments with your healthcare team, including your primary care physician, endocrinologist, and other specialists as needed. Discuss your diabetes management goals, review your progress, and address any concerns or questions you may have about your health.

Creating Your Personalized Wellness Plan:

Assess Your Current Health: Start by evaluating your current health status, including your blood sugar levels, diet, physical activity levels, stress levels, and medication regimen. Identify areas for improvement and set specific goals for each aspect of your wellness plan.

Establish Achievable, Specific, Measurable, Attainable, Relevant, and Time-Bound Objectives (SMART): Establish realistic, attainable goals. To keep yourself motivated and monitor your development over time, break down more ambitious goals into smaller, more doable tasks.

Seek Support: Don't hesitate to reach out to healthcare professionals, support groups, or online communities for guidance, encouragement, and support. Surround yourself with a supportive network of friends, family, and healthcare providers who can help you stay on track with your wellness plan.

Stay Flexible: Be flexible and open to making adjustments to your wellness plan as needed based on your progress, changing circumstances, and feedback from your healthcare team. Remember that managing diabetes is a lifelong journey, and it's okay to adapt your approach over time.

Creating a personalized diabetes wellness plan is essential for effectively managing the condition and promoting overall health and well-being. By incorporating strategies such as dietary modifications, physical activity, stress management, blood sugar monitoring, medication management, and regular medical check-ups, individuals can take control of their diabetes and live a healthier, more fulfilling life. By including diabetes-friendly teas as part of their wellness plan, individuals can enjoy additional health benefits and support their overall diabetes management goals.

CONCLUSION

One major theme that has come out of this in-depth investigation of diabetes treatment is the priceless contribution tea makes to the general health and wellbeing of diabetics. We have covered a wide range of subjects under the heading "Diabetes Tea Recipes," from the science underlying tea's effect on blood sugar regulation to the varied selection of herbal tea recipes designed especially for the management of diabetes. As we conclude our conversation, it is important to consider the role that tea plays as a comprehensive tool in the treatment of diabetes and what it means for people who want to have the best possible health.

First and foremost, our exploration has highlighted the various health benefits of tea consumption in the context of diabetes management. From green tea's rich antioxidant content to the anti-inflammatory properties of turmeric tea, each type of tea offers unique advantages that can complement traditional diabetes management strategies. For example, the polyphenols found in green tea have been shown to improve insulin sensitivity and reduce the risk of developing type 2 diabetes, making it a valuable addition to the diet of individuals at risk for the condition. Similarly, the cinnamon-infused warmth of cinnamon tea has demonstrated potential in lowering blood sugar levels, offering a flavorful alternative for those seeking to add variety to their diabetes-friendly beverages.

Moreover, our exploration has underscored the importance of mindfulness and holistic approaches in diabetes management. Tea rituals, such as mindful tea drinking and incorporating tea into meditation practices, serve as powerful tools for reducing stress levels and promoting relaxation.

As stress is known to adversely affect blood sugar control, integrating these mindful practices into daily life can have profound implications for diabetes management, fostering a sense of calm and balance amidst the challenges of living with the condition.

Additionally, our discussion has emphasized the significance of personalized wellness plans in diabetes management. By tailoring lifestyle choices to individual needs and preferences, individuals can create sustainable strategies for achieving optimal health outcomes. Whether it involves crafting a balanced diet, engaging in regular physical activity, or developing stress management techniques, a personalized approach enables individuals to take ownership of their health and empower themselves to make informed decisions about their diabetes care.

Furthermore, the concept of "Diabetes Tea Recipes" extends beyond mere beverage recommendations; it embodies a holistic philosophy of self-care and empowerment. By embracing the art of tea preparation and consumption, individuals can cultivate a deeper connection with their bodies and minds, fostering a sense of well-being that transcends the physical realm. Whether sipping on a soothing cup of chamomile tea before bedtime or enjoying the invigorating aroma of ginger tea in the morning, each tea ritual becomes a moment of mindfulness and self-reflection, guiding individuals on their journey towards better health and vitality.

In conclusion, the journey of diabetes management is not one-size-fits-all but rather a dynamic and multifaceted exploration of individual needs and preferences. Through the lens of "Diabetes Tea Recipes," we have embarked on a journey of discovery, uncovering the therapeutic potential of tea in supporting blood sugar regulation, promoting relaxation, and enhancing overall well-being. As individuals continue to navigate the complexities of living with diabetes, may they find solace and inspiration in the simple yet profound act of brewing a cup of tea—a moment of nourishment for the body, mind, and soul.

Thank you for taking the time to explore the world of "Diabetes Tea Recipes" with us. We hope this journey has been both enlightening and inspiring as we've uncovered the therapeutic potential of tea in managing diabetes and promoting overall well-being. By incorporating diabetes-friendly teas into your daily routine, you're not only savoring delicious flavors but also nurturing your body and mind in a holistic way. Cheers to your health and wellness, and may your tea-drinking adventures continue to enrich your life.

www.ingramcontent.com/pod-product-compliance
Lightning Source LLC
Chambersburg PA
CBHW050802260726
48660CB00004B/1201